CURRICULUM DEVELOPMENT FOR MEDICAL EDUCATION

CURRICULUM DEVELOPMENT FOR MEDICAL EDUCATION

A SIX-STEP APPROACH

David E. Kern, M.D., M.P.H.

Associate Professor of Medicine
The Johns Hopkins University School of Medicine
Co-Director, Division of General Internal Medicine
Johns Hopkins Bayview Medical Center
Baltimore, Maryland

Patricia A. Thomas, M.D.

Assistant Professor of Medicine
Deputy Director for Education, Department of Medicine
The Johns Hopkins University School of Medicine
Division of General Internal Medicine
Johns Hopkins Hospital
Baltimore, Maryland

Donna M. Howard, R.N., Dr.P.H.

Assistant Professor of Medicine
Curriculum Development and Evaluation Coordinator
Faculty Development Program for Clinician-Educators
The Johns Hopkins University School of Medicine
Division of General Internal Medicine
Johns Hopkins Bayview Medical Center
Baltimore, Maryland

Eric B. Bass, M.D., M.P.H.

Associate Professor of Medicine
Director, General Internal Medicine Fellowship Program
The Johns Hopkins University School of Medicine
Division of General Internal Medicine
Johns Hopkins Hospital
Baltimore, Maryland

THE JOHNS HOPKINS UNIVERSITY PRESS / BALTIMORE AND LONDON

The Johns Hopkins University Press
2715 North Charles Street, Baltimore, Maryland 21218-4363
www.press.jhu.edu

A catalog record for this book is available from the British Library.

Library of Congress Cataloging-in-Publication Data

Curriculum development for medical education:
a six-step approach/David E. Kern . . . [et al.].
p.   cm.
Includes bibliographical references and index.
ISBN 0-8018-5844-5 (pbk. : alk. paper)
1. Curriculum planning. 2. Medical education—
United States—Curricula. 3. Medicine—Study
and teaching. I. Kern, David E.
[DNLM: 1. Curriculum. 2. Education,
Medical—methods. W 18 C975 1998]
R834.C87 1998
610'.71'173—dc21
DNLM/DLC for Library of Congress
97-51745 CIP

To the many faculty members
who strive to improve medical education
by developing, implementing, and evaluating
curricula in the health sciences.

Contents

Acknowledgments

The authors wish to acknowledge the many medical educators who have contributed ideas and examples for this book. We thank Dr. Randy Barker, Dr. Norman Jensen, and Dr. Jack Ende, in particular, for reviewing and providing feedback on the book and its approach to curriculum development and evaluation. We thank our families for tolerating the many hours we have devoted to the production of this book. Finally, we acknowledge the excellent typographic assistance of Ms. Susan McFeaters in preparing numerous revisions of the manuscripts for this book.

CURRICULUM DEVELOPMENT FOR MEDICAL EDUCATION

Introduction

PURPOSE

The purpose of this book is to provide a practical, theoretically sound approach to developing, implementing, evaluating, and continually improving educational experiences in medicine.

TARGET AUDIENCE

This book is designed for use by program directors and others who are responsible for the educational experiences of students, residents, fellows, and clinical practitioners. It should be particularly helpful to those who are beginning or are in the midst of developing a curriculum.

DEFINITION OF THE CURRICULUM

In this book, a curriculum is defined as *a planned educational experience.* This definition encompasses a breadth of educational experiences, from one or more sessions on a specific subject, to a clinical rotation or clerkship, to an entire training program.

RATIONALE FOR THE BOOK

It is the responsibility of program directors and other medical faculty to plan educational experiences, often without having received training or acquired experience in such endeavors, and often in the presence of limited resources and significant institutional constraints. Recently, the Accreditation Council for Graduate Medical Education in the United States and its Residency Review Committees began to require written curricula (1).

Ideally, medical education should change as our knowledge base changes and as the needs, or the perceived needs, of patients, medical practitioners, and society change. Some contemporary demands for change and curriculum development are listed in Table I.1. This book assumes that medical educators will benefit from learning a practical, generic, and timeless approach to curriculum development that can address today's as well as tomorrow's needs.

BACKGROUND

The approach described in this book has evolved over the past 11 years, during which time the authors have taught curriculum development and evaluation skills to 101

Table I.1.   Some Contemporary Demands for Medical Education

Generic Demands
- Integrate principles of clinical epidemiology, clinical decision making, evidence-based medicine, and cost-effectiveness into all clinical training.
- Emphasize a patient-centered, problem-oriented, as opposed to a disease-oriented, approach in clinical training.
- Emphasize a holistic, biopsychosocial approach in most clinical training, rather than separate the biomedical from the psychosocial components of care.
- Train primary care physicians in population- and community-centered, as well as person-centered, approaches to providing health care.
- In recognition of the constantly evolving nature of medical knowledge and the impossibility of imparting a complete knowledge base, set of skills, or pattern of practice to trainees, focus the content of training on what is most relevant today, train physicians as effective problem solvers who can efficiently access an ever-evolving medical knowledge base, and motivate physicians to become effective, self-directed, lifelong learners.
- In recognition of the increasing complexity of medical care delivery, train physicians as managers and team members.
- Help physicians become proficient in recognizing and managing personal feelings, beliefs, values, and needs that can subconsciously affect their relations with patients and others (self-awareness).
- Increase the quantity and quality of clinical training in ambulatory, same-day surgery, subacute care, and chronic care settings, and reduce the amount of training in inpatient services of acute hospitals, as necessary to meet training needs.
- Train the number of primary care physicians and specialty physicians required to meet societal needs.
- Certify competence in procedures.
- Develop faculty to meet the above demands.

Demands for Specific Curricula
- Clinical epidemiology and decision making
- Informatics
- Interviewing/communication/patient education skills
- Behavioral/psychosocial medicine
- Management and team skills
- Preventive medicine
- Nutrition
- Geriatrics
- Training in new surgical (e.g., video-assisted, minimally invasive) techniques for practicing surgeons
- Primary care–oriented residency programs
- Specific curricula for primary care physicians
  Dermatology
  Gynecology
  Musculoskeletal medicine
  Ophthalmology
  Otolaryngology
  Minor surgery
  Practice management
  Environmental/occupational medicine
- Teaching and curriculum development skills for clinician-educators

faculty and fellows in the Johns Hopkins University Faculty Development Program for Clinician-Educators. Participants in the program's 10-month-long Curriculum Development Workshop have developed and implemented 42 medical curricula, in topics as diverse as advance directives, office gynecology for the generalist, a renal elective for internal medicine residents, and an office-based preceptorship for first-year medical students.

OVERVIEW OF BOOK

Chapter 1 presents an overview of a six-step approach to curriculum development. Chapters 2 through 7 describe each step in detail. Chapter 8 discusses how to maintain and improve curricula over time. Chapter 9 discusses how to disseminate curricula within and beyond institutions.

Throughout the book, *examples* are provided to illustrate major points. Most examples come from the real-life curricular experiences of the authors or their colleagues but may have been adapted for the sake of brevity or clarity. Some examples are taken from the literature; those that are fictitious were designed to be realistic and to demonstrate an important concept or principle.

Chapters 2 through 9 end with *questions* that encourage the reader to review the principles discussed in each chapter and to apply them to a desired, intended, or existing curriculum. These chapters include, in addition to the list of *specific references* that are cited in the text, an annotated list of *general references* that can guide the reader who is interested in pursuing a particular topic in greater depth.

Appendix A provides examples of curricula that have progressed through all 6 steps, and Appendix B supplements the chapter references by providing the reader with a selected list of published and unpublished resources for funding, faculty development, and already-developed curricula. At the end of the book, there is an *evaluation sheet,* which we hope you will return, so that the next edition of this book (if there is one) can meet the needs of our readers even better than this edition.

REFERENCE

1. American Medical Association. Section II. Essentials of accredited residencies in graduate medical education: Institutional and program requirements. In *Graduate Medical Education Directory, 1998–1999.* Chicago, Ill.: American Medical Association; 1998. Pp. 25–341.

Overview: A Six-Step Approach to Curriculum Development

RATIONALE AND ORIGINS

The six-step approach described in this book derives from the generic approaches to curriculum development set forth by Taba (1), Tyler (2), Yura and Torres (3), and others (4) and from the work of McGaghie et al. (5) and Golden (6), who advocate the linking of curricula to health care needs. Underlying assumptions are: (a) educational programs have aims or goals, whether or not they are clearly articulated; (b) medical educators have a professional and ethical obligation to meet the needs of their learners, patients, and society; (c) medical educators should be held accountable for the outcomes of their interventions; and (d) a logical, systematic approach to curriculum development will help achieve these ends.

A SIX-STEP APPROACH (FIGURE 1.1)

Step 1: Problem Identification and General Needs Assessment

The first step begins with the *identification and critical analysis of a health care need or other problem.* The need may relate to a specific health problem, such as the provision of care to patients infected with human immunodeficiency virus (HIV), or to a group of problems, such as the provision of routine gynecologic care by primary care physicians. It may relate to qualities of the physician, such as the need for health care providers to develop as self-directed, lifelong learners who can provide effective care as medical knowledge and practice evolve. Or it may relate to the health care needs of society in

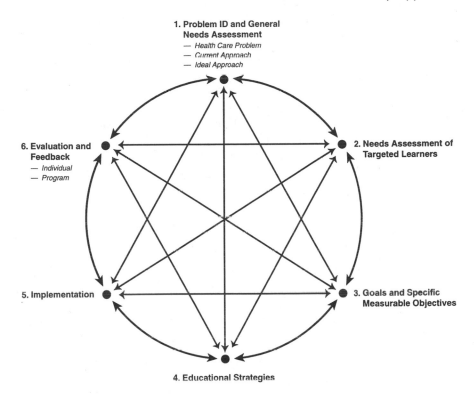

Figure 1.1.   A Six-Step Approach to Curriculum Development

general, such as whether the quantity and type of physicians being produced are appropriate.

A complete problem identification requires an analysis of the *current approach* of patients, practitioners, the medical education system, and society, in general, to addressing the identified need. This is followed by the identification of an *ideal approach,* which describes how patients, practitioners, the medical education system, and society should be addressing the need. The difference between the ideal approach and the current approach represents a *general needs assessment.*

Step 2: Needs Assessment of Targeted Learners

This step involves assessing the needs of one's targeted group of learners or medical institution, which may be different from the needs of learners and medical institutions in general.

EXAMPLE: The *general needs assessment of practicing primary care physicians* may have revealed (a) deficits in their provision of acute and preventive care to HIV-infected patients; (b) biases against homosexual and substance-abusing patients, resulting in avoidance of such patients; and (c) the lack of formal training. The *needs assessment of one's targeted learners,* however, may reveal that all of these learners have received training and feel comfortable caring for patients with HIV disease in the hospital, and that they almost all feel comfortable providing care for homosexual patients. On the other hand, these learners may have received no training and may exhibit deficits in the preventive care of HIV-infected patients and may have negative feelings about caring for patients who are substance abusers. Accordingly, new curriculum development for these learners would best focus on preventive care and on barriers to caring for substance-abusing HIV-infected patients.

Step 3: Goals and Objectives

Once the needs of targeted learners have been identified, goals and objectives for the curriculum can be written, starting with *broad or general goals,* then moving to *specific, measurable objectives.* Objectives may include cognitive (knowledge), affective (attitudinal), or psychomotor (skill and performance) objectives for the learner, process objectives related to the conduct of the curriculum, or even clinical outcome objectives. Goals and objectives are crucial because they help to determine curricular content and learning methods and help to focus the learner. They facilitate communication of what the curriculum is about to others and provide a basis for its evaluation. When resources are limited, prioritization of objectives can expedite the rational allocation of those resources.

Step 4: Educational Strategies

Once objectives have been clarified, *curriculum content is chosen and educational methods are selected that will most likely achieve the educational objectives.*

EXAMPLE: *Curriculum Content.* Based upon the above example of a needs assessment of targeted learners, one objective of this HIV curriculum might be to help targeted learners become proficient in the use of antiretroviral agents. Curriculum content, therefore, will need to focus on antiretroviral agents and their appropriate use.

EXAMPLES: *Educational Methods.* Case-based, problem-solving exercises that actively involve the learners are more likely to improve clinical reasoning skills than is attendance at lectures.

The development of physicians as effective team members is more likely to be achieved through their participating in and reflecting on cooperative learning experiences and work environments than through reading and discussing a book on the subject.

Interviewing, physical examination, and procedural skills will be best learned in an environment that supplements practice with self-observation, observation by others, feedback, and reflection.

Step 5: Implementation

Implementation of a curriculum has *several components:* procurement of political support for the curriculum; identification and procurement of resources; identification and address of barriers to implementation; introduction of the curriculum (e.g., piloting the curriculum on a friendly audience before presenting it to all targeted learners, phasing in the curriculum one part at a time); administration of the curriculum; and refinement of the curriculum over successive cycles. *Lack of attention to any of these components can threaten the success of a curriculum.*

Step 6: Evaluation and Feedback

This last step has several components. It usually is desirable to assess the performance of both *individuals* (individual evaluation) and the *curriculum* (called program evaluation). The purpose of evaluation may be *formative* (to provide ongoing feedback so that the learners or curriculum can improve) or *summative* (to provide a final "grade" or assessment of the performance of the learner or curriculum).

Evaluation can be used not only to drive the ongoing learning of participants and the improvement of a curriculum but also to gain support and resources for a curriculum, and, in research situations, to answer questions about the effectiveness of a specific curriculum or the relative merits of different educational approaches.

THE INTERACTIVE AND CONTINUOUS NATURE OF THE SIX-STEP APPROACH

In practice, curriculum development does not usually proceed in sequence, one step at a time. Rather, it is a dynamic, interactive process. Progress is often made on two or more steps simultaneously. Progress on one step influences progress on another (as illustrated by the bidirectional arrows in Figure 1.1). For example, limited resources (Step 5) may restrict the number and nature of objectives (Step 3) as well as the extent of evaluation (Step 6) that is possible. The development of evaluation methods (Step 6) may result in a refinement of objectives (Step 3). Evaluation (Step 6) may also provide information that serves as a needs assessment of targeted learners (Step 2). Time pressures, or the presence of an existing curriculum, may result in the development of goals, educational methods, and implementation strategies (Steps 3 and 4) prior to a formal problem identification and needs assessment (Steps 1 and 2), so that Steps 1 and 2 are used to refine and improve an existing curriculum rather than develop a new one.

For a successful curriculum, curriculum development never really ends, as illustrated by the circle in Figure 1.1. Rather, the curriculum evolves, based upon evaluation results, changes in resources, changes in targeted learners, and changes in the material requiring mastery.

REFERENCES

1. Taba H. *Curriculum Development: Theory and Practice.* New York: Harcourt, Brace, and World; 1962. Pp. 1–515.
2. Tyler RW. *Basic Principles of Curriculum and Instruction.* Chicago; University of Chicago Press; 1950. Pp. 1–83.
3. Yura H, Torres GJ, eds. *Faculty-Curriculum Development: Curriculum Design by Nursing Faculty.* New York: National League for Nursing; Publication No. 15-2164, 1986. Pp. 1–371.
4. Sheets KJ, Anderson WA, Alguire PC. Curriculum development and evaluation in medical education: Annotated bibliography. *J Gen Intern Med* 1992; 7(5):538–543.
5. McGaghie WC, Miller GE, Sajid AW, Telder TV. *Competency-Based Curriculum Development in Medical Education: An Introduction.* Geneva: World Health Organization; 1978. Pp. 1–99.
6. Golden AS. A model for curriculum development linking curriculum with health needs. In Golden AS, Carlson DG, Hogan JL, eds., *The Art of Teaching Primary Care.* New York: Springer Publishing; 1982. Pp. 9–25.

CHAPTER TWO

Step 1: Problem Identification and General Needs Assessment

DEFINITIONS

The first step in designing a curriculum is to *identify and characterize the health care problem* that will be addressed by the curriculum, how it is currently being addressed, and how it should be addressed. The difference between how the health care problem is currently being addressed, in general, and how it should be addressed is called a *general needs assessment*. Because the difference between the current and ideal approaches can be considered part of the problem that the curriculum will address, Step 1 is sometimes referred to, simply, as *problem identification*.

IMPORTANCE

The better a problem is defined, the easier it will be to design an appropriate curriculum to address the problem, because all the other steps in the curriculum development process depend on having a clear understanding of the problem (see Figure 1.1). Step 1 (problem identification and general needs assessment) and Step 2 (needs assessment of targeted learners) are particularly helpful in focusing a curriculum's goals and objectives (Step 3), which in turn help focus the curriculum's educational and evaluation strategies (Steps 4 and 6).

IDENTIFICATION OF THE HEALTH CARE PROBLEM

The ultimate purpose of a curriculum in medical education is to address a problem that affects the health of the public or a given population (1–3). Frequently, the problem of interest is a complex one with many facets. Even the simplest health problem, however, may be refractory to any educational or other intervention, if the problem has not been well defined. A comprehensive definition of the problem should include consideration of the epidemiology of the problem, as well as the impact of the problem on patients, health care professionals, and society (Table 2.1).

In defining the problem of interest, it is important to explicitly identify *whom* the problem affects. Does the problem affect a group of people with a particular disease (e.g., frequent disease exacerbations requiring hospitalization in patients with asthma)? Or does the problem affect society at large (e.g., irrational fears about the risk of transmitting the human immunodeficiency virus)? Does the problem directly or indirectly affect health professionals and their trainees (e.g., physicians inadequately prepared to provide ambulatory care or teach in the ambulatory setting)? Does the problem affect health care organizations or other corporate entities (e.g., failure to practice cost-effective medicine)? In many cases, the problem of interest may affect many different groups. The approximate number of people affected by the problem has implications for curriculum development, because a problem that affects a large number of people may warrant more attention than a problem that affects a relatively small number of people. Knowledge of who is affected by the problem, and knowledge of the characteristics and behaviors of those affected, is needed to guide decisions about the most appropriate target audience for a curriculum, the formulation of learning objectives, and the development of curriculum content.

Once those who are affected by the problem have been identified, it is important to elaborate *what* the effects on these people are. What is the effect of the problem on clinical outcomes, quality of life, quality of health care, use of health care and other re-

Table 2.1.   Identification and Characterization of the Health Care Problem

Whom does it affect?
    Patients
    Health care professionals
    Society

What does it affect?
    Clinical outcomes
    Quality of life
    Quality of health care
    Use of health care and other resources
    Medical and nonmedical costs
    Patient and provider satisfaction
    Work and productivity
    Societal function

What is the *quantitative and qualitative importance* of the effects?

Table 2.2.   The General Needs Assessment

What is *currently* being done by the following?
    Patients
    Health care professionals
    Medical educators
    Society

What personal and environmental factors affect the problem?
    Predisposing
    Enabling
    Reinforcing

Ideally, what should be done by the following?
    Patients
    Health care professionals
    Medical educators
    Society

What are the key *differences* between the current and ideal approaches?

sources, medical and nonmedical costs, patient and provider satisfaction, work and productivity, and the functioning of society? In describing these effects, their quantitative and qualitative importance should be considered.

GENERAL NEEDS ASSESSMENT (TABLE 2.2)

Current Approach

Having defined the nature of the health care problem, the next task is to assess current efforts to address the problem. The process of determining the current approach to a problem is sometimes referred to as a "job analysis" (1), which can be viewed as an assessment of the "job" that is currently being done to deal with a problem. To determine the current approach to a problem, the curriculum developer should ask what is being done by the following:

a. Patients
b. Health care professionals
c. Medical educators
d. Society

Knowledge of what *patients* are and are not doing to address a problem may influence decisions about curriculum content. For example, are patients using noneffective treatments or engaging in activities that exacerbate a problem—behaviors that need to be reversed? Or are patients predisposed to engage in activities that could alleviate the problem—behaviors that need to be encouraged?

Knowledge of how *health care professionals* are currently addressing the problem is especially relevant, because they are usually the target audience for medical curricula.

EXAMPLE: More than one million persons in the United States are infected with human immunodeficiency virus (HIV). Individuals with HIV infection receive health care from primary care practitioners and from infectious disease specialists. Studies may suggest that infectious disease specialists achieve better outcomes for their HIV-infected patients than do primary care practitioners by making the most appropriate use of available medications. However, there may not be enough infectious disease specialists to care for all the people who have HIV infection. Given this information, a curriculum on primary care of HIV-infected patients should address the issue of how primary care practitioners can remain up to date on the appropriate use of new medications.

Most of the problems that are important enough to warrant development of a focused curriculum are problems that are being encountered and addressed in many different places. For this reason, it is wise to explore what is currently being done by other *medical educators* to help patients and health care professionals address the problem. Clearly, much can be learned from the previous work of educators who have tried to tackle the problem of interest. For example, patient education materials and classes as well as curricula for medical students, residents, practicing physicians, and other health care professionals may already be in existence and may be of great value in developing a curriculum for one's own target audience. A dearth of relevant curricula will reinforce the need for innovative curricular work.

While curriculum developers are usually not in the position to bring about societal change, it is important to be cognizant of what *society* is doing to address the problem.

EXAMPLE: In designing a curriculum to help health care professionals reduce the spread of HIV infection in a given society, it is useful to know how the society handles the distribution of condoms and clean needles.

In understanding the current approach to addressing a health problem, it is useful to consider *personal and environmental factors* that may aggravate or alleviate the problem. Factors that can influence the problem can be classified as predisposing factors, enabling factors, or reinforcing factors (4). *Predisposing factors* refers to knowledge, attitudes, and beliefs of people that influence their motivation to change (or not to change) behaviors related to a problem. *Enabling factors* generally refers to personal skills and societal or environmental forces that may help or hinder efforts to change a problem behavior. *Reinforcing factors* refers to the various types of feedback, including rewards and punishments, that encourage continuation or discontinuation of a desired or undesired behavior. Identification of the environmental factors should include assessment of organizational, administrative, and political factors that may influence the problem.

EXAMPLE: In designing a curriculum for family practice residents on the prevention of smoking-related illness, curriculum developers identified important personal and environmental factors that influence an individual's smoking behavior. These factors included an individual's self-defined readiness to quit; an individual's health concerns and beliefs regarding self and family; an individual's sense of personal efficacy or empowerment; an individual's personal experiences related to smoking; attitudes and behaviors of family, friends, and peers; societal prohibitions, as in restaurants, on airplanes, or at workplaces; societal economic factors; societal messages, such as advertisements and government warnings; availability of cigarettes, cigars, and pipe tobacco; costs of smoking; strength of physical and psychological addiction; personally defined benefits to smoking; personally defined motivators for stopping or not starting; and personally defined barriers to cessation. These factors were considered in designing a recommended approach for residents' participation in a school health program and for counseling individual pediatric, adolescent, and adult patients about smoking and smoking cessation.

By considering all aspects of how a health problem is addressed, one can determine the most appropriate role for an educational intervention in addressing the problem, keeping in mind the fact that an educational intervention by itself usually cannot solve all aspects of a complex health problem.

Ideal Approach

Having determined the current approach to the problem, the next task is to determine the ideal approach to the problem. The process of determining the ideal approach to a problem is sometimes referred to as a "task analysis," which can be viewed as an assessment of the specific "tasks" that need to be performed to appropriately deal with the problem (1, 5). To determine the ideal approach to a problem, the curriculum developer should ask what each of the following groups should do to deal most effectively with the problem:

a. Patients
b. Health care professionals
c. Medical educators
d. Society at large

In determining the ideal approach to a problem, it is helpful to determine the extent to which *patients* should be involved in handling the problem themselves.

> **EXAMPLE:** An educational program that is designed to prevent atherosclerotic cardiovascular disease should address patient understanding of and compliance with effective preventive behaviors related to diet, exercise, smoking, and the use of over-the-counter medications.

With respect to *health care professionals,* it is helpful for the curriculum developer to decide *which* professionals should deal with the problem and *what* they should be doing. Answering these questions can help curriculum developers choose or confirm their choice of targeted learners and decide upon the appropriate content for a curriculum. If more than one type of health care professional typically encounters the problem, it is necessary to decide whether it is appropriate for all practitioners to handle the problem or whether it might be better to have some practitioners refer the problem to practitioners who have greater expertise in handling the problem.

> **EXAMPLE:** Family physicians and internists routinely manage many common gynecologic problems. They, or the system in which they work, must decide which patients, with what specific problems, should be referred to a gynecologist.

Determining the ideal approach for *medical educators* involves identifying the appropriate target audiences, the appropriate content, the best educational strategies, and the best evaluation methods to ensure effectiveness.

While curriculum developers usually are not in the position to effect *societal* change, it is important to realize that some of their targeted learners may be in such a position now or in the future. A curriculum, therefore, may choose to address not only current environmental or societal factors that contribute to a problem but also those environmental and societal changes that might alleviate the problem.

EXAMPLE: Some residents who took part in a curriculum on violence became involved in local and national efforts to reduce the prevalence of domestic and gun-related violence.

The ideal approach should serve as an important, but not rigid, guide to developing a curriculum. One needs to be flexible in accommodating others' views and the many practical realities related to curriculum development. For this reason, it is useful to identify the basis for one's "ideal" approach: individual opinion, consensus, the logical application of established theory, or scientific evidence. Obviously, one should be more flexible with respect to an "ideal" approach based upon individual opinion than to an "ideal" approach based upon scientific evidence.

Differences between Current and Ideal Approaches

Having determined the current and ideal approaches to a problem, the curriculum developer should identify the differences between the two approaches, termed a *general needs assessment.* These differences should be the main target of any plans for addressing the health care problem.

OBTAINING THE NECESSARY INFORMATION

Many methods can be used to identify and characterize a health care problem and to determine the current and ideal approaches to that problem (1–3). The most commonly used methods are listed in Table 2.3.

The curriculum developer should start with a *well-focused review of information that is already available.* A medical librarian can be extremely helpful in accessing the medical and relevant nonmedical (e.g., educational) literature, as well as in accessing the increasing number of computerized databases that contain relevant, but unpublished, information.

A *review of the medical literature,* including journal articles and textbooks, is generally the most efficient method for gathering available information about a health care problem and about what is currently being done to deal with it, as well as what should be done to deal with it. In reviewing the literature on a clinical topic, it is important to look for pertinent clinical practice guidelines because the guidelines may clearly delineate the ideal approach to a problem. Recently, there has been a tremendous proliferation of clinical practice guidelines, covering a wide variety of clinical issues, so it is quite likely that curriculum developers will be able to find one or more guidelines for a clinical problem of interest. Sometimes guidelines conflict in their recommendations. It is necessary to critically appraise the methods used to develop the guidelines in order to determine which recommendations should be included in one's ideal approach (6, 7).

Other sources of available information also should be considered, especially when the published literature is sparse (see Appendix B, Additional Resources). Occasionally, *reports by professional societies or governmental agencies* can provide relevant information about a problem. *Curriculum documents submitted to educational clearinghouses, obtained directly from funding agencies or other institutions,* or *accessed through the Internet* (8), can be particularly helpful to the curriculum developer by providing specific examples of what is being done by other medical educators to address a problem.

Table 2.3.   Methods for Obtaining the Necessary Information

Review of Available Information
    Published literature
    Reports by professional societies or government agencies
    Documents submitted to educational clearinghouses
    Curriculum documents from other institutions
    Patient education materials prepared by foundations or professional organizations
    Public health statistics
    Clinical registry data
    Administrative claims data

Use of Consultants/Experts
    Informal consultation
    Formal consultation
    Meetings of experts

Collection of New Information
    Surveys of patients, practitioners, or experts
    Focus group(s)
    Nominal group technique
    Group-mailed delphi technique
    Daily diaries by patients and practitioners
    Observation of tasks performed by practitioners
    Time and motion studies
    Critical incident reviews
    Study of ideal performance cases or role model practitioners

EXAMPLE: An example of one database of educational material is the Educational Clearinghouse for Internal Medicine developed by the Association of Program Directors in Internal Medicine (see Appendix B: Additional Resources). This database includes a wide variety of educational documents and materials that have been prepared by educators from many institutions.

In some cases, it may be worthwhile to contact *colleagues at other institutions* who are performing related work and who may be willing to share information that they have developed or collected. For some health problems, *patient education materials* have been prepared by foundations or professional organizations, and these materials can provide information about the problem from the patient's perspective, as well as material to use in one's curriculum.

Public health statistics, clinical registry data, and *administrative claims data* can be used for obtaining information about the incidence or prevalence of a problem. Most medical libraries will have reports on the vital statistics of the population, which are published by the federal government. Clinical registry data may be difficult to access directly, but reports from clinical registries can be identified by searching the medical literature on a particular clinical topic. In the United States, the federal government and many states maintain administrative claims databases that provide data on the use of inpatient and outpatient medical services. Such data can help to define the magnitude of a clinical problem. Because of the enormous size of most claims databases, special expertise is needed to perform analyses of such data (9). Despite their potential value in defining a problem, these types of databases rarely have the depth of information that is needed to guide curriculum planning.

Even though the curriculum developer may be expert in the area to be addressed by the curriculum, it is frequently necessary to ask other experts how they interpret the information about a problem, particularly when the available literature gives conflicting information. In such cases, *expert opinions* can be obtained by informal or formal consultation or by organizing a meeting of experts to discuss the issues. For most curricula, this can be done on a relatively informal basis with local experts. Occasionally, the problem is so controversial or important that the curriculum developer may wish to spend the additional time and effort necessary to obtain formal input from outside experts.

When the available information about a problem is so inadequate that curriculum developers cannot draw reasonable conclusions, it is desirable to *collect new information* about the problem. *In-person interviews* with a small sample of patients, students, practitioners, medical educators, or experts can yield information relatively quickly, but may or may not be representative. Such interviews may be conducted individually or in the format of a *focus group* of 8 to 12 people where the purpose is to obtain in-depth views regarding the topic of concern (10, 11). Obtaining consensus of the group is not the goal; rather it is to elicit the range of perspectives regarding it. Another small-group method occasionally used in needs assessment is the *nominal group technique,* which employs a structured, sometimes iterative, approach to identifying issues, solutions, and priorities (12). The outcome of this technique is an extensive list of brainstormed and rank-ordered ideas. Yet another method is the *small-group or modified Delphi technique,* which employs an iterative process not only to generate ideas or answers to a question but also to move a group toward consensus (13).

Often the most convenient way to collect new information about a problem is to perform a *survey* (14) by mail (15) or telephone (16). The *mailed Delphi technique* is a special iterative survey technique that uses the same panel of respondents over time and feeds back group responses to respondents on each successive cycle in order to promote consensus (13).

More-intensive methods of data collection include the *use of daily diaries* (17) by practitioners or patients, *observation by work sampling* (1, 2) (which involves direct observation of a sample of patients, practitioners, or medical educators in their work settings), *time and motion studies* (1, 18) (which involves observation and detailed analysis of how patients and/or practitioners spend their time), *critical incident reviews* (1, 2, 19, 20) (wherein cases having desired and undesired outcomes are reviewed to determine how the process of care relates to the outcomes), and *review of ideal performance cases.* These latter methods require considerable time and resources but may be valuable in selected instances where detailed information is needed about a particular aspect of clinical practice.

Regardless of what methods are used to obtain information about a problem, it is necessary to synthesize that information in an efficient manner. A logical, well-organized report, with tables that summarize the collected information, is one of the most common methods for accomplishing the synthesis. A well-organized report has the advantages of efficiently communicating this information to others as well as being available for quick reference in the future. Collected reference materials and resources can be filed for future access. A less common, but useful, method for synthesizing information related to a specific aspect of a problem is the use of a fishbone diagram (21) (see example below).

EXAMPLE: A number of methods could be used to determine the current and ideal approaches to training physicians to address the ethical aspects of clinical decision making in ambulatory settings. A literature review should be conducted but may not yield much information about issues that have been raised by recent developments in the managed care industry. Experts could be consulted; they may have strong opinions about how ethical dilemmas should be handled but may lack objective information on how their recommended approaches affect outcomes such as patient satisfaction. In this situation, it would be valuable to collect information by interviewing or surveying a sample of patients and practitioners from a variety of managed care organizations. Information that might be obtained from such a process could be summarized in a fishbone diagram:

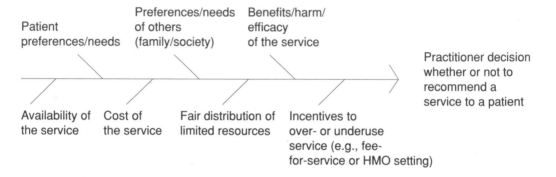

TIME AND EFFORT

Those involved in the development of a curriculum must decide how much they are willing to spend, in terms of time, effort, and other resources, for problem identification and general needs assessment. Too little time and effort runs the risk of having a curriculum that is poorly focused and unlikely to address adequately the problem of concern. Too much time and effort runs the risk of leaving insufficient resources for the other steps in the curriculum development process. Careful consideration of the nature of the problem is necessary to achieve an appropriate balance.

Some problems are complex enough to require a great deal of time in order to adequately understand them. On the other hand, problems that have been less well studied previously may require more time and effort than problems that have been well studied, because original data may need to be collected for the less-studied problems.

One of the goals of this step is for the curriculum developer to become enough of an expert in the area to make decisions about curricular objectives and content. The curriculum developer's prior knowledge of the problem area, therefore, will also determine the amount of time and effort he or she needs to spend on this step.

The time and effort spent on defining the problem of interest may yield new information or new perspectives that warrant publication in the medical literature (see Chapter 9: Dissemination). However, the methods employed in the problem identification and general needs assessment must be rigorously applied and described if the results are to be published in a peer reviewed journal. The curriculum developer must decide whether the academic value of such a publication is worth the time and effort that would be diverted from the development of the curriculum itself.

Time pressures, or the inheritance of an existing curriculum, may result in a situation in which the curriculum is developed prior to an adequate problem identification and general needs assessment. In such situations, a return to this step may be very helpful in explaining or improving an existing curriculum.

CONCLUSION

By clarifying the health care problem that a curriculum hopes to address, and the current and ideal approaches to addressing the problem, it may become apparent that a curriculum per se cannot solve all aspects of the problem, particularly if the problem is a complex one. Nevertheless, this clarification is essential in helping the curriculum developer focus an educational intervention so that the intervention can make a contribution to solving the problem.

It is important to keep in mind that the conclusions drawn from the general needs assessment may or may not apply to the particular group of learners targeted by a curriculum developer. For this reason, it is also necessary to perform an explicit assessment of the specific needs of one's targeted learners (see Chapter 3) before proceeding with further development of a curriculum.

QUESTIONS

For the curriculum you are coordinating, planning, or would like to be planning, please consider the following:

1. Identify a health care problem that is (will be) addressed by this curriculum.

2. *Whom* does the problem affect?

3. *What* effects does the problem have on these people?

4. How important is the problem, *quantitatively and qualitiatively?*

5. Based upon your current knowledge, use the top row of the table below to list some of the things that patients, health care professionals, educators, and society at large are doing *currently* to address the problem.

	Patients	Health Care Professionals	Medical Educators	Society
Current [Approach]				
Ideal [Approach]				

6. Based upon your current knowledge, use the bottom row of the table above to list key things that patients, health care professionals, educators, and society should *ideally* be doing to address the problem.

7. Perform a *general needs assessment* by identifying the differences between the current and ideal approaches.

8. Identify key areas in which your knowledge has been deficient for this exercise. Given your available resources, what *methods* would you use to correct these deficiencies? (See Table 2.3.)

GENERAL REFERENCES

Golden AS. A model for curriculum development linking curriculum with health needs. In Golden AS, Carlson DG, Hogan JL, eds., *The Art of Teaching Primary Care.* Springer Series on Medical Education, vol. 3. New York: Springer Publishing Co.; 1982. Pp. 9–25.
   This chapter addresses the role of task and job analysis in the development of competency-based curricula.

Green LW, Kreuter MW. *Health Promotion Planning: An Educational and Environmental Approach.* Mountain View, Calif.: Mayfield Publishing Co.; 1991.
   This work provides a sound conceptual basis for developing plans to change health behaviors. 506 pages.

Witkin BR, Altschuld JW. *Planning and Conducting Needs Assessments: A Practical Guide.* Thousand Oaks, Calif.: Sage Publications; 1995.
   This work provides a detailed discussion of how to plan and conduct a needs assessment. 302 pages.

SPECIFIC REFERENCES

1. Golden AS. A model for curriculum development linking curriculum with health needs. In Golden AS, Carlson DO, Hogan JL, eds., *The Art of Teaching Primary Care.* Springer Series on Medical Education, vol. 3. New York: Springer Publishing Co.; 1982. Pp. 9–25.
2. McGaghie WC, Miller GE, Sajid AW, Telder TV. *Competency-Based Curriculum Development in Medical Education: An Introduction.* Geneva: World Health Organization; 1978. Pp. 21–41.
3. Harden RM. Ten questions to ask when planning a course or curriculum. *Med Educ* 1986; 20:356–365.
4. Green LW, Kreuter MW. *Health Promotion Planning. An Educational and Environmental Approach.* Mountain View, Calif.: Mayfield Publishing Co.; 1991. Pp. 22–31.
5. Arsham GM, Colenbrander A, Spivey BE. A prototype for curriculum development in medical education. *J Med Educ* 1973; 48:78–84.
6. Hayward RSA, Wilson MC, Tunis SR, Bass EB, Guyatt GH. Users' guides to the medical literature. VIII. How to use clinical practice guidelines. Part A. Are the results valid? *JAMA* 1995; 274:570–574.
7. Wilson MC, Hayward RSA, Tunis SR, Bass EB, Guyatt GH. Users' guides to the medical literature: VIII. How to use clinical practice guidelines. Part B. What are the recommendations, and will they help you in caring for your patients? *JAMA* 1995; 274:1630–1632.
8. Peters R, Sikorski R. Navigating to knowledge: Tools for finding information on the Internet. *JAMA* 1997; 277:505–506.

9. Romanov PS, Luft HS. Getting the most out of messy data: Problems and approaches for dealing with large administrative data sets. In Geady ML, Schwartz H. eds., *Medical Effectiveness Research Data Methods*. Rockville, Md.: U.S. Department of Health and Human Services, 1992 AHCPR Publication No. 92-0056. Pp. 57–75. [just these pages]

10. Krueger RA. *Focus Groups: A Practical Guide for Applied Research.* Newbury Park, Calif.: Sage Publications; 1988.

11. Stewart DW, Shamdasani PN. *Focus Groups: Theory and Practice,* Applied Social Research Methods Series, vol. 20. Newbury Park, Calif.: Sage Publications; 1990.

12. Witkin BR, Altschuld JW. *Planning and Conducting Needs Assessments: A Practical Guide.* Thousand Oaks, Calif.: Sage Publications; 1995. Pp. 167–171.

13. Witkin BR, Altschuld JW. *Planning and Conducting Needs Assessments: A Practical Guide.* Thousand Oaks, Calif.: Sage Publications; 1995. Pp. 193–203.

14. Fink A. *How to Ask Survey Questions.* Thousand Oaks, Calif.: Sage Publications; 1995.

15. Bourque LB, Fielder EP. *How to Conduct Self-Administered and Mail Surveys.* Thousand Oaks, Calif.: Sage Publications; 1995.

16. Frey JH, Oishi SM. *How to Conduct Interviews by Telephone and in Person.* Thousand Oaks, Calif.: Sage Publications; 1995.

17. Denzin NK, Lincoln YS, eds., *Handbook of Qualitative Research.* Thousand Oaks, Calif.: Sage Publications; 1994. Pp. 205, 224, 287, 463.

18. Timm PR, Stead JA. *Communication Skills for Business and Professions.* Upper Saddle River, N.J.: Prentice Hall; 1996. Pp. 638.

19. Witkin BR, Altschuld JW. *Planning and Conducting Needs Assessments: A Practical Guide.* Thousand Oaks, Calif.: Sage Publications; 1995. Pp. 150–151.

20. Flanagan JC. The critical incident technique. *Psychological Bulletin* 1954; 51:327–358.

21. Witkin BR, Altschuld JW. *Planning and Conducting Needs Assessments: A Practical Guide.* Thousand Oaks, Calif.: Sage Publications; 1995. Pp. 243–249.

CHAPTER THREE

Step 2: Needs Assessment of Targeted Learners

DEFINITION

A *needs assessment of targeted learners* is a process by which curriculum developers identify the *differences between the ideal and the actual characteristics of the targeted learner group and between the ideal and actual characteristics of their environment.*

IMPORTANCE

The needs of a curriculum's targeted learners, whether they are patients, practitioners, practitioners in training, or students, are likely to be somewhat different from the needs of learners in general. A curriculum's targeted learners may already be proficient in one area of general need but have particular learning needs in another area. Unless curriculum developers assess the needs of their targeted learners, their curriculum may be inefficient, on the one hand, because the curriculum devotes unnecessary resources to areas the learners have already mastered, and ineffective, on the other, because the curriculum has devoted insufficient resources to areas of particular need.

EXAMPLE: Curriculum developers planning an ethics curriculum for PGY-2 and -3 residents during an ambulatory medicine rotation reviewed previous curricula to which the residents had been exposed in the residency, spoke individually to several residents, and surveyed all targeted residents about their previous training, perceived competencies, and perceived needs. The developers discovered that the residents had been exposed to considerable training related to autonomy, beneficence, substitute judgment, advance directives, and end-of-life decisions, but not at all to clinical decision making in the context of competing interests such as patient versus family versus societal needs, or managed care versus fee-for-service incentives. All of the residents' training had centered around inpatient cases. The curriculum developers, therefore, decided to focus their curriculum on clinical decision making, with an emphasis on the ambulatory setting.

IDENTIFICATION OF TARGETED LEARNERS

Before curriculum developers can proceed with the needs assessment of targeted learners, they must identify their targeted learners. Ideally this choice of targeted learners would flow from the problem identification and general needs assessment. The targeted learners would be the group most likely, with further learning, to contribute to the solution of the problem. Frequently, however, curriculum developers have already been assigned their targeted learners, such as medical students or resident physicians in training. In this case, it is worth considering whether an educational intervention directed at one's targeted learners could contribute to solving the health care problem of concern.

CONTENT

The first step in the needs assessment of targeted learners, once they have been identified, is to decide upon the information that is most needed. Such information might include: previous and already planned training and experiences; existing proficiencies; current performance; perceived deficiencies and needs; learning styles, preferences, and experiences regarding different learning strategies; barriers, enabling factors, and reinforcing factors (see Chapter 2) in the environment in which the targeted learners learn and apply the learning; and resources available to the learners (Table 3.1). The problem identification and general needs assessment can be used to target the information in each area that is most relevant to the curriculum being developed. Curriculum developers may already have some of this information; other information may have to be acquired.

METHODS

General Considerations

When the desired information about the targeted learners is not already known by the curriculum developers, they must decide how to acquire it. As with problem identification and general needs assessment, curriculum developers must decide *how much time, effort, and resources should be devoted to this step.* Too little time and effort risks development of an inefficient or ineffective curriculum. Too much time and effort can diminish the resources available for other critical steps, such as the development of effective educational strategies, successful implementation of the curriculum, and evaluation. Since resources are almost always limited, the curriculum developers will need to *prioritize* their information needs.

Table 3.1.   Content Potentially Relevant to a Needs Assessment of Targeted Learners

- Previous training and experiences relevant to the curriculum
- Already-planned training and experiences relevant to the curriculum
- Existing proficiencies
    - Cognitive: knowledge; problem-solving abilities
    - Affective: attitudes, values, beliefs, role expectations
    - Psychomotor skills: history, physical examination, procedures, counseling
- Current performance
- Perceived deficiencies and learning needs
- Preferences and experiences regarding different learning strategies
    - Time
    - Format
    - Methods
- Characteristics of the learners' and the curriculum's environment
    - Barriers
    - Enabling factors
    - Reinforcing factors
- Resources available to learners
    - Patients and clinical experiences
    - Information resources
    - Computers
    - Audiovisual equipment
    - Role models, teachers, mentors
    - Other

Once the information that is required has been decided upon, the curriculum developers should decide what is the *best method, given limited resources,* to obtain this information. In making this decision, they should ask the following questions: What *standards of representativeness and accuracy* will be required? Will *subjective or objective, quantitative or qualitative data* be preferable?

> **EXAMPLE:** If there is strong disagreement within the group responsible for developing the curriculum about the knowledge, attitude, skill, or performance deficits of the targeted learners, a more rigorous, representative, objective, and quantitative assessment of learner needs may be required.

> **EXAMPLE:** In-depth qualitative data gathered from a sample of selected learners and faculty may be most useful to a curriculum developer who is new to an institution.

If the curriculum developers have limited or no experience in using a needs assessment method, it is wise to seek *advice or mentorship from those with expertise* in the method. Before applying a method formally to the group of targeted learners, it is important to *pilot* the data collection instrument on a convenient, friendly audience.

> **EXAMPLE:** A questionnaire was developed to assess the perceived learning needs and preferences of a targeted group of resident physicians. It was piloted on a few friendly residents and faculty, one with expertise in survey methodology. Feedback from the pilot revealed that the questionnaire was too long and that some of the questions were worded in a confusing

manner. Feedback provided specific suggestions on improved wording and format, on what questions could be cut, and on one new question that the curriculum developers decided to add. If the original questionnaire had been sent out without revision, much of the data would have been unusable.

Specific Methods

Specific methods commonly used in the needs assessment of targeted learners include: informal discussion or formal interviews with individual learners or their supervisors or observers; small group or focus group discussions with proposed participants in the curriculum; questionnaires; direct observation of targeted learners; pretests of knowledge, attitudes, or skills; audits of current performance; and strategic planning sessions for the curriculum (1–4). The advantages and disadvantages of each method are displayed in Table 3.2. Data already in existence, such as the results of standardized examinations (e.g., national board, in-service, and specialty board examinations), procedure and experience logs, other curricula to which the targeted learners are exposed, and audit results, may provide information relevant to curriculum developers and may obviate the need for independent data collection.

RELATION TO OTHER STEPS

The information one chooses to collect as part of the needs assessment of targeted learners may be influenced by what one expects will be a *goal* or *objective* of the curriculum, or by the *educational and implementation strategies* being considered for the curriculum. *Goals and objectives, educational strategies, implementation, and evaluation* are likely to be affected by what is learned in the needs assessment of targeted learners. The process of conducting a needs assessment can serve as advance publicity for a curriculum and can ease its *implementation.* Information gathered as part of the *needs assessment of targeted learners* can serve as "*pre,*" or "*before,*" data for evaluation of the effect of a curriculum. In this case curriculum developers may insist on higher methodologic standards than would be necessary for the needs assessment alone. For all of these reasons, it is wise to think through other steps, at least in a preliminary manner, before investing time and resources in the needs assessment of targeted learners.

> **EXAMPLE:** A needs assessment of targeted learners revealed barriers in terms of space, equipment, and support staff, as well as skill deficits, that prevented residents from including cervical cancer screening in the care of their ambulatory continuity patients. The curriculum developers were able to convince the clinic administrator to purchase the necessary equipment and to redefine nursing staff roles with respect to availability for pelvic examinations. Space needs were incorporated into planning for the new ambulatory building.

> **EXAMPLE:** On the first day of a curriculum, learners were administered a knowledge and problem-solving test. They performed better than expected in some areas and not as well as expected in other areas. This information was used to tailor subsequent learning sessions. Test data were used as part of a pre-post evaluation of the learners' cognitive achievements in the curriculum.

It is also worth noting that one can learn a lot about a curriculum's targeted learners in the course of conducting the curriculum. This information can then be used as a needs assessment of targeted learners for the next cycle of the curriculum.

Table 3.2.   Advantages and Disadvantages of Different Needs Assessment Methods

Method	Advantages	Disadvantages
Informal discussions	Convenient Inexpensive Rich in detail and qualitative information	Lack of methodologic rigor Variations in questions Interviewer biases
Formal interviews	Standardized approach to interviewee Methodologic rigor possible Questions and answers can be clarified With good response rate, can obtain data representative of entire group of targeted learners Quantitative and/or qualitative information	Methodologic rigor requires trained interviewers and measures of reliability Costly in terms of time and effort, especially if methodologic rigor required Interviewer bias and influence on respondent
Focus group discussions	Efficient method of "interviewing" several at one time Group interaction may enrich or deepen information obtained Qualitative information	Requires skilled facilitator to control group interaction and minimize facilitator influence on responses Views of quiet participants may not be expressed No quantitative information Information may not be representative of all targeted learners
Questionnaires	Standardized questions Methodologic rigor relatively easy With good response rate, can obtain representative data Quantitative and/or qualitative information Can assess affective traits (attitudes, beliefs, feelings)	Requires skill in writing clear, unambiguous questions Answers cannot be clarified or developed Requires time and effort to ensure methodologic rigor and response rate Requires time, effort, and skill to construct valid tests of affective traits
Direct observation	Best method for assessing skills Can be informal or methodologically rigorous Informal observations can sometimes be accomplished as part of one's teaching or supervisory role	Can be time-consuming, especially if methodologic rigor desired Guidelines must be developed for standardized observations Observer bias Impact of observer on observed Assesses ability, not real-life performance (unless observations are unobtrusive)

Table 3.2.   (*continued*)

Method	Advantages	Disadvantages
Tests	Efficient, objective means of assessing cognitive or psychomotor abilities Tests of key knowledge items relatively easy to construct	Requires time, effort, and skill to construct valid tests of skills and higher-order cognitive abilities Test anxiety may affect performance Assesses ability, not real-life performance
Audits of current performance	Useful for medical record keeping and provision of recorded care (e.g., tests ordered, provision of discrete preventive care measures, prescribed treatments) Unobtrusive Assesses real-life performance Can be methodologically rigorous with standards, instructions, and ensurance of inter- and intra-rater reliability	Requires development of standards Requires resources to pay and train auditors, time and effort to perform audit oneself Recording omissions Indirect, incomplete measure of care
Strategic planning sessions for the curriculum*	Can involve targeted learners as well as key faculty Can involve brainstorming of learner needs as well as of current program strengths and weaknesses Can involve prioritization as well as generation of needs Creates sense of involvement and responsibility in participants Part of a larger process that also identifies goals, objectives, and responsibilities	Requires skilled facilitator to ensure participation and lack of inhibition by all participants Requires considerable time and effort to plan and conduct successful strategic planning sessions and to develop the associated report

*Strategic planning (2–4) is a team-building process that involves key individuals in the brainstorming and discussion of existing strengths and weaknesses; the brainstorming, discussion, and prioritization of needs, goals, and objectives; the assignment of responsibilities; and the establishment of timetables.

EXAMPLE: During an ambulatory medicine rotation, it was noted that residents were, for the most part, unskilled in incorporating preventive care into office visits and in motivating patients to follow treatment plans. Focused training in these areas was developed for the next cycle of ambulatory medicine rotations.

CONCLUSION

By clarifying the specific needs of one's targeted learners, the curriculum developer can help assure that the curriculum being planned not only addresses important general needs, but also is relevant to the specific needs of its learners. Steps 1 and 2 provide a sound basis for the next step, choosing the goals and objectives for the curriculum.

QUESTIONS

For the curriculum you are coordinating, planning, or would like to be planning, please consider the following:

1. *Identify your targeted learners.* From the point of view of your problem identification and general needs assessment, will training this group, as opposed to other groups of learners, make the greatest contribution to solving the health care problem? If not, who would be a better group of targeted learners? Are these learners an option for you? Notwithstanding these considerations, is it nevertheless important to train your original group of targeted learners? Why?

2. To the extent of your current knowledge, *describe your targeted learners and their environment* in terms of existing proficiencies, current performance, attitudes, previous and already planned training, learning needs, enabling and reinforcing factors and barriers in the learners' environment, familiarity and preferences regarding different learning methods, and resources for learning.

3. *What information* about your learners and their environment *is unknown* to you? *Prioritize* your information needs.

4. *Identify one or more methods* by which you could obtain the most important information. For each method, *identify the resources* (time, personnel, supplies, space) required to develop the necessary data collection instruments and to collect and analyze the needed data. To what degree do you feel each method is feasible?

5. Identify individuals upon whom you could *pilot* your needs assessment instrument(s).

GENERAL REFERENCES

Green LW, Kreuter MW, Deeds SG, Partridge KB. *Health Education Planning: A Diagnostic Approach.* Palo Alto, Calif.: Mayfield Publishing; 1980.
This work is a basic text in health education program planning that includes the importance and role of the needs assessment in determining a social/quality-of-life diagnosis and in identifying health problems [epidemiologic diagnosis] for a targeted population. 306 pages.

Rossett A. *Training Needs Assessment*. Englewood Cliffs, N.J.: Educational Technology Publications; 1987.

> This is a practical book that focuses on determining the training needs of employees in organizations, with concepts, examples, and needs assessment methods that are easily transferable to all levels of healthcare workers and professionals. The book is written from an instructional design perspective with good references from that field. 294 pages.

Windsor R, Baranowski T, Clark N, Cutter G. *Evaluation of Health Promotion and Education Programs*. Palo Alto, Calif.: Mayfield Publishing; 1984.

> This work is a basic text in the evaluation of health programs, starting with the importance of sound program planning, including needs assessment as the process by which "what is and what ought to be" are identified and measured. 366 pages.

Witkin BR, Altschuld JW. *Planning and Conducting Needs Assessments: A Practical Guide*. Thousand Oaks, Calif.: Sage Publications; 1995.

> This is a readable yet comprehensive book with information and examples organized in two major sections: (1) planning and managing the needs assessment, and (2) methods used for conducting a needs assessment. The methods section is particularly useful. It covers records and social indicators (including mapping); surveys; interviews; the critical incident technique; nominal group technique; focus groups; mailed Delphi survey and modified (or group) Delphi process; strategic planning; and causal analysis, including fishboning, cause-and-consequence analysis, and fault tree analysis. The organizational and community examples are easily translatable to medical care settings. 302 pages.

SPECIFIC REFERENCES

1. Witkin BR, Altschuld JW. *Planning and Conducting Needs Assessments: A Practical Guide*. Thousand Oaks, Calif.: Sage Publications; 1995. Pp. 101–274.
2. Witkin BR, Altschuld JW. *Planning and Conducting Needs Assessments: A Practical Guide*. Thousand Oaks, Calif.: Sage Publications; 1995. Pp. 210–217.
3. Barry BW. *Strategic Planning Workbook for Nonprofit Organizations*. St. Paul, Minn.: Amherst H. Wilder Foundation; 1986. P. 72.
4. Goodstein LD, Nolan TM, Pfeiffer JW. *Applied Strategic Planning: An Introduction*. San Diego, Calif.: Pfeiffer and Co.; 1992. P. 61.

Additional references on specific methods are cited in Chapter 2 under "Obtaining the Necessary Information."

Step 3: Goals and Objectives

DEFINITIONS

Once the needs of the learners have been clarified, it is desirable to target the curriculum to address these needs by setting goals and objectives. *A goal or objective is defined as an end toward which an effort is directed.* In this book, the term *goal* will be used when a *broad educational objective* is being discussed. The term *objective* will be used when a *specific measurable objective* is being discussed.

> **EXAMPLE:** A *goal,* or *broad educational objective,* of a gynecology curriculum for internal medicine residents might be that internal medicine residents develop the knowledge, attitudes, and skills necessary to diagnose, manage, and appropriately refer women who present to primary care settings with gynecologic needs or complaints. A *specific measurable objective* of the curriculum might be that, by the end of the gynecology curriculum, each resident will have demonstrated, at least once, the appropriate technique, as defined on a check sheet, for obtaining a Pap smear and cervical cultures.

IMPORTANCE

Goals and objectives are important because they do the following:

- Help direct the choice of curricular content and the assignment of relative priorities to various components of the curriculum
- Suggest what learning methods will be most effective
- Enable evaluation of learners and the curriculum, thus permitting demonstration of the effectiveness of a curriculum

- Suggest what evaluation methods are appropriate
- Clearly communicate to others (e.g., to learners; faculty; residency directors, department chairs, and others with administrative responsibility; and individuals from other institutions) what the curriculum addresses and hopes to achieve

Broad educational goals communicate the overall purposes of a curriculum and serve as criteria against which the selection of various curricular components can be judged. The development and prioritization of *specific measurable objectives* permit further refinement of the curricular content and guide the selection of appropriate educational and evaluation methods.

WRITING OBJECTIVES

Writing educational objectives is an underappreciated skill. Learners, teachers, and curriculum planners frequently have difficulty in formulating or explaining the objectives of a curriculum despite the importance of objectives.

A key to writing useful educational objectives is to make them *specific* and *measurable.* Such objectives should contain *five basic elements* (1): <u>Who</u> <u>will do</u> <u>how much</u> <u>(how well)</u> <u>of what</u> <u>by when</u>? (<u>Who</u> is the first element, <u>will do</u> is the second, <u>how much</u> or <u>how well</u> is the third, <u>of what</u> is the fourth, and <u>by when</u> is the fifth.)

> **EXAMPLE:** The example provided at the beginning of the chapter contains these elements: Who (each resident) will do (demonstrate, obtain) how much (once) of what (the appropriate technique for a Pap smear and cervical cultures) by when (the end of the curriculum). That objective could be measured by observation using a checklist.

In writing specific measurable objectives (as opposed to goals), one should *use words that are open to few interpretations* (e.g., to list or demonstrate) rather than words that are open to many interpretations (e.g., to know or be able). Table 4.1 provides lists of more- and less-precise words to use in writing objectives. Finally, *it is important to have persons who are not involved in the curriculum review the objectives,* to ensure that others can accurately describe what the objectives are intended to convey. Some examples of poorly written and better written objectives are provided in Table 4.2.

TYPES OF OBJECTIVES

In constructing a curriculum, one should be aware of the different types and levels of objectives. *Types of objectives* include objectives related to the achievements of *learners,* to the educational *process* itself, and to health care and other *outcomes* of the curriculum. These types of objectives can be written at the *level* of the *individual* learner and at the level of the *program* or of all learners in *aggregate.* Table 4.3 provides examples of each type and level of objective for a curriculum on smoking cessation.

Learner Objectives

Learner objectives include objectives that relate to learning in the cognitive, affective, and psychomotor domains. Learner objectives that pertain to the *cognitive* domain of learning are often referred to as "knowledge" objectives. The latter terminology, however, may lead to an overemphasis on factual knowledge. Objectives related to the cog-

Table 4.1.   Words Open to More and Fewer Interpretations

Words Open to More Interpretations	Words Open to Fewer Interpretations
know or understand	list
	recite
	present
	sort, distinguish
	define
	describe
	give an example of
be able	demonstrate (as measured by)
know how	
internalize	use or incorporate into performance (as measured by)
appreciate	rate as valuable
grasp the significance of	rank as important
believe	identify, rate, or rank as a belief or opinion
enjoy	rate or rank as enjoyable
learn	(Use one of the above terms.)
teach	(Use one of the above terms; do not confuse the teacher and the learner in writing learner objectives.)

nitive domain of learning should take into consideration a spectrum of cognitive functioning relevant to the goals of a curriculum, from simple factual knowledge to higher levels of cognitive functioning, such as problem solving and clinical decision making.

> **EXAMPLE:** *Cognitive Objective.* By the end of the neurology curriculum, the learner will describe in writing a cost-effective approach to the initial evaluation and management of patients with dementia (an approach that includes at least six of the eight elements listed on their handout).

Learner objectives that pertain to the *affective* domain are frequently referred to as "attitudinal" objectives. They may refer to specific attitudes, values, beliefs, biases, emotions, or role expectations that can affect learning or performance. Affective objectives are usually more difficult to express and measure than cognitive objectives are (2). Many people, therefore, are uncomfortable with writing affective objectives in explicit terms, even though affective objectives are implicit in most educational programs for medical students, physicians, and other providers. To the extent that a curriculum involves learning in the affective domain, curriculum planners should develop objectives in this domain. Such objectives can help direct educational strategies, even when there are insufficient resources to objectively assess their achievement.

> **EXAMPLE:** *Affective Objective.* By the end of the HIV curriculum, all residents will have identified their attitudes and beliefs regarding HIV patients who are drug addicts and will have discussed with their colleagues and attending physicians how these might influence their management of such patients.

Table 4.2. Examples of Less-Well-Written and Better-Written Objectives

Less-Well-Written Objectives	Better-Written Objectives
▪ Residents will learn the techniques of joint injections. [*The types of injections to be learned are not specified. The types of residents are not specified. It is unclear whether cognitive understanding of the technique is sufficient or whether skills must be acquired. It is unclear by when the learning must have occurred and how proficiency could be assessed. The objective on the right addresses each of these concerns.*]	▪ By the end of their residency, each family practice resident will have demonstrated at least once (according to the attached protocol) the proper techniques of: —subacromial, bicipital, and intra-articular shoulder injection; —intra-articular knee aspiration and/or injection; —injections for lateral and medial epicondylitis; —injections for deQuervain's tenosynovitis; and —aspiration and/or injection of at least one new bursa, joint, or tendinous area, using appropriate references and supervision.
▪ By the end of their internal medicine clerkship, each third-year medical student will be able to diagnose and manage common ambulatory medical disorders. [*This objective specifies "who" and "by when" but is vague about what specifically the medical students are to achieve. The two objectives on the right add specificity to the latter.*]	▪ By the end of their internal medicine ambulatory clerkship, each third-year medical student will have achieved cognitive proficiency in the diagnosis and management of hypertension, diabetes, angina, chronic obstructive pulmonary disease, hyperlipidemia, alcohol and drug abuse, smoking, and asymptomatic HIV infection, as measured by acceptable scores on interim tests and the final examination. • By the end of their internal medicine clerkship, each third-year medical student will have seen and discussed with their preceptor, or discussed in a case conference with colleagues, at least one patient with each of the above disorders.
▪ Physician practices whose staff complete the three-session communication skills workshops will have more satisfied patients. [*This objective does not specify the comparison group or what is meant by "satisfied." The objective on the right specifies more precisely which practices will have more satisfied patients, what the comparison group will be, and how satisfaction will be measured. It specifies one aspect of performance as well as satisfaction. One could look at the satisfaction questionnaire and the telephone management monitoring instrument for a more precise description of the outcomes being measured.*]	▪ Physician practices that have ≥50% of their staff complete the three-session communication skills workshops will have lower complaint rates, higher patient satisfaction scores on the yearly questionnaire, and better telephone management as measured by random simulated calls than practices that have lower completion rates.

Table 4.3.   Types and Levels of Objectives. Examples from a Smoking Cessation Curriculum for Residents

	Level of Objective	
	Individual Learner	Aggregate or Program
LEARNER Cognitive (Knowledge)	By the end of the curriculum, each resident will be able to list the 8-step approach to effective smoking cessation counseling.	By the end of the curriculum, ≥80% of residents will be able to list the 8-step approach to effective smoking cessation counseling, and ≥90% will be able to list the 4 critical (asterisked) steps.
Affective (Attitude)	By the end of the curriculum, each primary care resident will rank smoking cessation counseling as an important and effective intervention by primary care physicians (≥3 on a 4-point scale).	By the end of the curriculum there will have been a statistically significant increase in how primary care residents rate the importance and effectiveness of smoking cessation counseling by primary care physicians.
Psychomotor (Skill or Competence)	During the curriculum, each primary care resident will demonstrate in role-play a smoking cessation counseling technique that incorporates the attached 8 steps.	During the curriculum, ≥80% of residents will have demonstrated in role-play a smoking cessation counseling technique that incorporates the attached 8 steps.
Psychomotor (Behavior or Performance)	By 6 months after completion of the curriculum, each primary care resident will have negotiated a plan for smoking cessation with ≥60% of his or her smoking patients or will have increased the percentage of such patients by ≥20% from baseline.	By 6 months after completion of the curriculum, there will have been a statistically significant increase in the % of GIM residents who have negotiated a plan for smoking cessation with their patients.
PROCESS	Each primary resident will have attended both sessions of the smoking cessation workshop.	≥80% of primary care residents will have attended both sessions of the smoking cessation workshop.
OUTCOME	By 12 months after completion of the curriculum, the smoking cessation rate (for ≥ 6 months) for the patients of each primary care resident will increase ≥2-fold from baseline or will be ≥10%.	By 12 months after completion of the curriculum, there will have been a statistically significant increase in the % of primary care residents' patients who have quit smoking (for ≥6 months).

Learner objectives that relate to the *psychomotor* domain of learning are often referred to as "skill" or "behavioral" objectives. These objectives refer to specific psychomotor tasks or actions that may involve hand or body movements, vision, hearing, speech, or the sense of touch. History taking, patient education, interpersonal communication, physical examination, record keeping, and procedural skills fall into this domain. In writing objectives for relevant psychomotor skills, it is helpful to indicate whether learners are only expected to achieve the ability to perform a skill (a "skill," or "competence," objective) or whether they are expected to incorporate the skill into their continuing behavior (a "behavioral," or "performance," objective). Whether a psychomotor skill is written as a competence or performance objective has important implications for the choice of evaluation strategies and may influence the choice of educational methods as well.

EXAMPLE: *Skill, or Competence, Objective.* By the end of the curriculum, all medical students will have demonstrated proficiency in assessing alcohol use by utilizing all four of the CAGE questions with one simulated and one real patient. (This skill, or competence, objective can be assessed by direct or videotaped observation by an instructor.)

EXAMPLE: *Behavioral, or Performance, Objective.* All students who have completed the curriculum will routinely (>80% of time) use the CAGE questions to assess their patients' alcohol use. (This behavioral, or performance, objective might be assessed by reviewing a random sample of student write-ups of the new patients whom they work up during their core medical clerkship.)

Often an objective includes elements from more than one domain. As long as the objective is clear, it is relatively unimportant how the objective is classified.

EXAMPLE: *Multidomain Objective.* In a curriculum on the psychosocial domain of medical care, one objective might be that, during the curriculum, each medical resident demonstrate the use of nonverbal cues from patients to diagnose depression. In this example, the recognition of nonverbal cues depends not only on knowledge of what nonverbal cues to look for but also on a complex set of interactive skills involving both vision and hearing. If the objective specified that residents routinely use these skills in clinical practice, then affective elements related to use, such as role perception and perceived efficacy, would also be involved.

Knowledge of the various domains of learner objectives is valuable because it helps one to understand the complexity of learning related to any educational goal and to choose objectives and educational strategies wisely.

Process Objectives

These objectives relate to the implementation of the curriculum. They may indicate the degree of participation that is expected from the learners. They may indicate the expected response of learners or faculty to a curriculum.

EXAMPLE: *Individual Process Objectives.* Each student in the orthopedics clerkship will spend at least three hours per day four days per week seeing patients in an ambulatory setting, spend at least 30 minutes of each session discussing cases with an attending physician, attend 90% or more of the scheduled didactic and case conferences, and present an evidence-based discussion on a clinical topic of their choice by the end of the clerkship.

EXAMPLE: *Program Process Objectives.* By the end of the clerkship, 90% or more of students will have completed and returned their evaluation forms. Eighty percent or more of students will recommend the clerkship to other students as an outstanding or good experience ("4" or "3" on a 4-point scale).

Outcome Objectives

Outcome objectives relate to potential outcomes, or effects, of a curriculum, beyond those delineated in its learner and process objectives. Outcomes might include health outcomes of patients or career choices of physicians. More proximal outcomes might include changes in the behaviors of patients or physicians. Sometimes a curriculum planner may choose to classify certain psychomotor (behavioral, or performance) objectives for learners as outcome objectives.

> **EXAMPLE:** *Career Outcome Objective.* Eighty percent or more of the graduates of our primary care residency programs will be pursuing careers in primary care five years after graduation.

> **EXAMPLE:** *Performance and Health Outcome Objectives.* Physicians who have completed the two-session, continuing education course on basic interviewing skills will demonstrate, during audiotaped doctor-patient encounters one to two months later, a significantly greater use of taught skills in their practice setting than control group physicians do. Their emotionally disturbed patients, as determined by General Health Questionnaire (GHQ) scores of 5 or more, will show significantly greater improvement in GHQ scores at two weeks, three months, and six months following the audiotaped encounters than patients of control group physicians (3).

It is often unrealistic to expect medical curricula to have easily measurable effects on quality of care and patient outcomes. (Medical students, e.g., may not have responsibility for patients until years after completion of a curriculum.) However, most medical curricula should be designed to have positive effects on quality of care and patient outcomes. Even if outcomes will be difficult or impossible to measure, the inclusion of some outcome objectives in a curriculum plan will emphasize the ultimate aims of the curriculum and may influence the choice of curricular content and educational methods.

> **EXAMPLE:** Including health outcome objectives for patients who present with a common problem may lead to emphasis in a curriculum on the content and clinical decision making skills that are expected to affect those patient outcomes.

At this point, it may be useful to review Table 4.3 once again for examples of each type and level of objective.

ADDITIONAL CONSIDERATIONS

While educational objectives are an important part of any curriculum, it is important to remember that *most educational experiences encompass much more than a list of preconceived objectives* (4, 5). For example, on clinical rotations much learning derives from unanticipated experiences with individual patients. In many situations, the most useful learning derives from learning needs identified and pursued by individual learners and their mentors. An exhaustive list of objectives in such settings can be overwhelming for learners and teachers alike, can stifle creativity, and can limit learning related to individual needs and experiences. On the other hand, if no goals or objectives are articulated, learning experiences will be unfocused, and important cognitive, affective, or psychomotor objectives may not be achieved.

Goals provide desired overall direction for a curriculum. An important and difficult task in curriculum development is to develop a *manageable number of specific measurable objectives* that do the following:

- Interpret the goals
- Focus and prioritize curricular components that are critical to the realization of the goals
- Encourage (or at least do not limit) creativity, flexibility, and nonspecified learning relevant to the curriculum's goals

> **EXAMPLE:** A broad goal for a residency in general internal medicine might be for learners to become proficient in the cost-effective diagnosis and management of common clinical problems. Once these clinical problems have been identified, patient case mix can be assessed to determine whether the settings used for training provide the learners with adequate clinical experience.
>
> Broad goals for clinical rotations in the same residency might be that residents develop as self-directed learners, develop sound clinical reasoning skills, and use patient centered approaches in the care they provide. Specific measurable process objectives could promote the achievement of these goals without being unnecessarily restrictive. One such objective might be that each resident, during the course of a one-month clinical rotation, present a 15-minute report on a patient management question encountered that month that incorporates principles of clinical epidemiology, clinical decision making, cost-effectiveness, and an assessment of patient or family preferences. A second objective might be that each resident do at least some targeted reading on each inpatient during the course of the month and briefly report, during rounds, on the sources used and on selected results of that reading.

Usually, several cycles of writing objectives are required to achieve a manageable number of specific measurable objectives that truly match the needs of one's targeted learners.

> **EXAMPLE:** Faculty developing a curriculum on diabetes for the residency in the above example might begin with the following objectives, that are to be achieved by the end of the curriculum:
>
> 1. Each resident will be able to list each complication of diabetes mellitus.
> 2. Each resident will be able to list atherosclerotic cardiovascular disease, retinopathy/blindness, nephropathy, neuropathy, and foot problems/amputation as complications of diabetes, and to list specific medical interventions that prevent each of these complications or their sequelae.
> 3. Each resident will be able to list all of the medical and sensory findings that are seen in each of the neuropathies that can occur as a complication of diabetes mellitus. (A similar objective might have been written for other complications of diabetes.)
> 4. Residents will know how to use insulin.
>
> After reflection and input from others, Objective #1 might be eliminated because remembering every complication of diabetes regardless of prevalence or management implications is felt to be of little value. Objective #3 might be eliminated because it requires detailed knowledge that is unnecessary for management by the generalist. Objective #4 might be rejected because it is too general and should be rewritten in specific measurable terms. Objective #2 might be retained because it is sufficiently detailed and relevant to the goal of training residents to be proficient in the cost-effective diagnosis and management of clinical problems commonly encountered in medical practice. In the above process, the curriculum team would have reduced the number of objectives while ensuring that the remaining objectives are sufficiently specific and relevant to direct and focus teaching and evaluation.

CONCLUSION

Writing goals and objectives is a critically important skill in curriculum development. Well-written goals and objectives define and focus a curriculum. They provide direction to curriculum developers in selecting educational strategies and evaluation methods.

QUESTIONS

For the curriculum you are coordinating, planning, or would like to be planning, please consider the following:

1. Write one to three broad educational goals.

2. Write one specific measurable educational objective of each type and at each level, using the template provided.

	Level of Objective	
	Individual Learner	Aggregate or Program
Learner (Cognitive, Affective, or Psychomotor)		
Process		
Outcome		

Check each objective to make sure that it includes all five elements of a specific measurable objective (<u>Who/will do/how much/of what/by when</u>?) Check to see that the words you used are precise and unambiguous (Table 4.1). Have someone else read your objectives and see if he or she can explain them to you accurately.

3. Do your specific measurable objectives support and further define your broad educational goals? If not, you need to reflect further on your goals and objectives and to change one or the other.

4. Reflect on how your objectives, as worded, will focus the content, educational methods, and evaluation strategies of your curriculum. Is this what you want? If not, you may want to rewrite, add, or delete some objectives.

GENERAL REFERENCES

Bloom BS. *Taxonomy of Educational Objectives: Cognitive Domain.* New York: Longman; 1984.
This classic text presents a detailed classification of cognitive educational objectives. A condensed version of the taxonomy is included in an appendix for quick reference. 207 pages.

Green L, Kreuter M, Deeds S, Partridge K. *Health Education Planning: A Diagnostic Approach.* Palo Alto, Calif.: Mayfield Publishing; 1980.
This basic text on health education program planning describes the role of objectives in program planning. 306 pages.

Gronlund NE. *How to Write and Use Instructional Objectives.* New York: MacMillan; 1991.
This comprehensive and well-written reference encompasses the cognitive, affective, and psychomotor domains of educational objectives. It provides a useful updating of Bloom's and Krathwohl's texts, with many examples and tables. 106 pages.

Krathwohl DR, Bloom BS, Masia BB. *Taxonomy of Educational Objectives: Affective Domain.* New York: Longman; 1964.
This classic text presents a detailed classification of affective educational objectives. A condensed version of the taxonomy is included in an appendix for quick reference. 196 pages

Mager RF. *Preparing Instructional Objectives.* Belmont, Calif.: David S. Lake, Publishers; 1984.
This is a readable, practical guide book for writing objectives. Examples are included. This book is a popular reference for professional educators as well as health professionals who develop learning programs for their students. 136 pages.

SPECIFIC REFERENCES

1. Green L, Kreuter M, Deeds S, Partridge K. *Health Education Planning: A Diagnostic Approach.* Palo Alto, Calif.: Mayfield Publishing; 1980. Pp. 48, 50, 64–65.
2. Henerson ME, Morris LL, Fitz-Gibbon CT. *How to Measure Attitudes* (book number 6). In Herman JL, ed., *Program Evaluation Kit.* Newbury Park, Calf.: Sage Publications; 1987. Pp. 9–13.
3. Roter DL, Hall JA, Kern DE, Barker LR, Cole KA, Roca RP. Improving physicians' interviewing skills and reducing patients' emotional distress: A randomized clinical trial. *Arch Intern Med* 1995; 155:1877–1884.
4. Ende J, Atkins E. Conceptualizing curriculum for graduate medical education. *Acad Med* 1992; 67:528–534.
5. Ende J, Davidoff F. What is curriculum? *Ann Intern Med* 1992; 116:1055–1057.

Step 4: Educational Strategies

DEFINITIONS

Once the goals and specific measurable objectives for a curriculum have been determined, the next step is to *develop the educational strategies* by which the curricular objectives will be achieved. Educational strategies involve both content and methods. *Content* refers to the specific material to be included in the curriculum. *Methods* refers to the ways in which the content is presented.

IMPORTANCE

Educational strategies provide the means by which a curriculum's objectives are achieved. They are the heart of the curriculum, the educational intervention itself. There is a natural tendency to think of the curriculum in terms of this step alone. As we shall see, the groundwork of Steps 1 through 3 guides the selection of educational strategies.

DETERMINATION OF CONTENT

The *content of the curriculum flows from its specific measurable objectives.* The amount of material presented to the learners should not be too little to lack substance or too much to overwhelm, and the material should not contain more detail than is necessary to achieve the desired objectives and outcomes. For some curricula, it is helpful to group or sequence objectives and their associated content in a manner that is logical and that promotes understanding. It is usually helpful to construct a *syllabus* for the curriculum that includes (a) an explicit statement of learning objectives and methods to help focus learners; (b) a schedule of the curriculum events and other practical information, such as locations and directions; (3) written curricular materials (e.g., readings, cases, questions); and (d) suggestions/resources for additional learning.

CHOICE OF EDUCATIONAL METHODS

General Guidelines (Table 5.1)

It is helpful to keep the following general principles in mind when considering educational methods for a curriculum:

- *Maintain Congruence between Objectives and Methods.* Choose educational methods that are most likely to achieve a curriculum's goals and objectives. One way to approach the selection of educational methods is to group the specific measurable objectives of the curriculum as cognitive, affective, or psychomotor objectives (see Chapter 4) and select educational methods most likely to be effective for the type of objective (see Table 5.2).

  EXAMPLE: *Cognitive Objective.* If an objective is to improve learners' higher cognitive skills, such as clinical decision making, then facilitated case discussions that involve learners are likely to be more effective than having a faculty member analyze the case for the learners.

  EXAMPLE: *Affective Objective.* If an objective is an attitudinal change, selected real-life experiences, combined with group discussion and reflection on the experiences, are more likely to achieve this goal than lectures or didactic pronouncements are.

  EXAMPLE: *Psychomotor Objective.* If an objective of a curriculum is to improve residents' ability to perform a procedure correctly, such as obtaining a PAP smear, supervised practice with feedback and discussion of performance is likely to be more effective than lectures about the technique.

- *Use Multiple Educational Methods.* Individuals have different preferences for learning, sometimes referred to as *learning styles* (1). Some prefer to hear information, others to have visual aids, and others tactile aids. Some learners thrive with organization and structure; others learn well in an unstructured environment where they discover what is to be learned. Medical students have been shown to have different motivations for learning, such as passing the course, understanding the material, or excelling, which affect the students' learning strategies or learning approaches (2). Ideally, the curriculum would use those methods that work best for individual learners. However, few curricula can be that malleable; often a large number of learners

Table 5.1. Guidelines for Choosing Educational Methods

- Maintain congruence between objectives and methods.
- Use multiple educational methods.
- Choose educational methods that are feasible in terms of resources.

Table 5.2.   Matching Educational Methods to Objectives

Education Method	Cognitive: Knowledge	Cognitive: Problem-Solving	Affective: Attitudinal	Psychomotor: Skills or Competence	Psychomotor: Behavioral or Performance
Readings	+++	+	+	+	
Lecture	+++	+	+	+	
Discussion	++	++	+++	+	+
Problem-solving exercises	++	+++	+		+
Programmed learning	+++	++		+	
Learning projects	+++	+++	+	+	+
Role models		+	++	+	++
Demonstration	+	+	+	++	++
Real-life experiences	+	++	++	+++	+++
Simulated experiences	+	++	++	+++	+
Audio or video review of learner	+			+++	+
Behavioral/ environmental interventions*			+	+	+++

Note: blank = not recommended; + = appropriate in some cases, usually as an adjunct to other methods; ++ = good match; +++ = excellent match (consensus ratings by authors).
* = removal of barriers to performance; provision of resources that promote performance; reinforcements that promote performance.

need to be accommodated in a short period of time. The use of different educational methods helps to overcome the problem of different learning styles. The use of different educational methods also helps to maintain *learner interest* and provides opportunities for *reinforcement of learning.* Such reinforcement can deepen learning, promote retention, and enhance the application of what has been learned.

The use of multiple educational strategies is particularly relevant in certain situations. For *curricula that attempt to achieve complex objectives spanning several domains* (see Chapter 4), the use of multiple educational methods is necessary to achieve congruence between objectives and methods. For *curricula that extend over longer time periods,* the use of multiple educational methods helps to maintain interest and reinforce previous learning.

EXAMPLE: A gynecology curriculum has as one objective that PGY-3 residents will perform 80% of screening PAP smears in their continuity clinic practices themselves. The curriculum includes knowledge-based *lectures* discussing cervical cancer risk, the importance of PAP smears, and compliance with screening by primary care physicians. Residents receive supervised training in the technique of PAP smears in a PGY-2 rotation (*experiential learning*). Their attitudes regarding the role of primary care physicians in screening for cervical cancer are discussed at the beginning and end of the curriculum (*discussion*). Yearly *audit* results are given to individual residents on their performance of PAP smears on their continuity practice patients.

- *Choose Educational Methods That Are Feasible in Terms of Resources.* Resource constraints may limit the implementation of the ideal approach in this step as well as in other steps. Curriculum developers will need to consider faculty time, space, availability of clinical material and experiences, and costs, as well as the availability of learner time. Faculty development may be an additional consideration, especially if an unfamiliar instructional method is chosen, such as role-play or the use of multimedia. Use of technology, such as computer-assisted learning, may involve initial cost but may save faculty resources over the time course of the curriculum. When resource limitations threaten the achievement of curricular outcomes, objectives and/or educational strategies (content and methods) will need to be further prioritized and selectively limited. The question then becomes, what is the most that can be accomplished, given the resource limitation?

In selecting education methods for a curriculum, it is helpful to consider the advantages and disadvantages of each method under consideration. Advantages and disadvantages of commonly used educational methods are summarized for the reader in Table 5.3. Specific methods are discussed below, in relation to their function.

Methods for Achieving Cognitive Objectives

Methods that are commonly used to achieve cognitive objectives include:

- Readings
- Lectures
- Audiovisual materials
- Discussion
- Programmed learning

The use of targeted *readings* can be an efficient method of presenting information and addressing cognitive objectives. The completion of readings, however, depends upon the presence of sufficient opportunity for learners to read and upon the motivation of individual learners. Existing publications may or may not efficiently target a curriculum's objectives. Learners can be directed to use readings more effectively if they are given explicit objectives and content for individual readings. A written syllabus can target specific educational objectives but requires faculty resources to construct it. Readings are commonly used to supplement other educational methods.

Perhaps the most universally applied method for addressing cognitive objectives is the *lecture,* which has as its advantages structure, low technology, and the ability to teach many learners in a short period of time. Successful lecturers develop skills that promote the learners' interest and acquisition of knowledge, such as controlling the physical environment, assessing and engaging the audience, organizing the material,

Table 5.3.   Summary of Advantages and Limitations of Different Educational Methods

Educational Method	Advantages	Disadvantages
Readings	Low cost Cover fund of knowledge Little preparation time	Passive learning Learners must be motivated to complete
Lectures	Low cost Accommodate large numbers of learners Structured presentation of complicated topics	Passive learning Teacher centered Quality depends on speaker/ audiovisual material
Discussion	Active learning Permits assessment of learner needs Allows learner to apply newly acquired knowledge Suitable for higher order cognitive objectives: problem solving and clinical decision making; can address affective objectives	More faculty intensive than readings or lectures Cognitive/experience base required of learners Group and facilitator dependent
Problem-based learning	Active learning Facilitates higher cognitive objectives: problem solving and clinical decision making; can incorporate objectives that cross domains: ethics, humanism, cost efficiency	Developmental costs Requires faculty facilitators and small groups Less efficient for transferring factual information
Programmed learning	Active learning Don't need clinical material at hand Safe simulations for learners Immediate feedback on knowledge, sequencing, efficiency, clinical decision making Learner applies new knowledge	Developmental costs if not commercially available May need computer access for learners if computer based
Learning projects	Active learning Promote, teach self-directed learning Learners set individual learning objectives Suitable for higher-order cognitive objectives	Learners need motivation Learners need basic skills to access learning resources Require effective faculty mentors

Table 5.3. (*continued*)

Method	Advantages	Disadvantages
Role models	Faculty often available Impact often seems profound	Require valid evaluation process to identify effective role models Specific interventions usually unclear Impact depends on interaction between specific faculty member and learner Outcomes multifactorial and difficult to assess
Demonstration	Efficient method for demonstrating skills/procedures	Passive learning Teacher centered Quality depends on speaker/audiovisual material
Artificial models	Safe environments to practice skills Learners can use at own pace; less faculty supervision required	May not be available for specific curriculum Can be expensive
Role plays	Suitable for objectives that cross domains: knowledge, attitudes, and skill Efficient Low cost Can be structured to be learner centered Safe environment for skills practice	Require trained faculty facilitators Learners need some basic knowledge or skills Can be resource intensive if large numbers of learners
Standardized patients	Ensure appropriate clinical material Approximate "real life" more closely than role plays Safe environment for skills practice Can give feedback to learners on performance Can be reused for ongoing curricula	Cost Requires expertise to develop and train SPs

Table 5.3.   (*continued*)

Method	Advantages	Disadvantages
Clinical experiences	"Real life" Promote learner motivation and responsibility Promote higher-level cognitive, attitudinal, skill, and performance learning	Require clinical material when learner is ready Require faculty to supervise and to provide feedback Learner needs basic knowledge or skill Need to be monitored for case mix, appropriateness Require reflection, follow-up
Audio or video reviews of learner	Provide accurate feedback on performance Provide opportunity for self-observation	Require trained faculty/facilitators Taping can be awkward or intrusive and pose logistical problems Require patient permission
Group learning	Active learning Resources usually available Allows multidisciplinary approaches Suitable for problem-based learning, clinical decision making, community-based projects Encourages cooperation, teamwork among learners	Group should have some training in group process skills, conflict management, etc. May require faculty facilitators with training in above Time required for successful functioning
Behavioral/ environmental interventions*	Influence performance	Assume competence Require control over learners' real-life environment

*Removal of barriers to performance; provision of resources that promote performance; reinforcements that promote performance.

making transitional and summary statements, presenting examples, using emphasis and selected repetition, effectively using audiovisual aids, and facilitating an effective question-and-answer period (3–6). The usual medical lecture is topic based, with the learners serving as passive recipients of information. The inclusion of problem-solving exercises or case discussions can engage the learners in a more active process that helps them to recognize what they may not know (i.e., to set learning objectives) and to apply new knowledge as it is learned.

Audiovisual materials are frequently used within the context of lectures, but can also be used in other contexts to reinforce content presented as readings or lectures. Clinic wall charts, wallet-sized flash cards, or computer reminders can reinforce items, such as preventive practice guidelines, discussed previously in greater depth. Videotapes can be used to present a lecture, when a lecturer is unavailable, or to conserve faculty resources when a lecture needs to be repeated many times. Videotapes can also be used to demonstrate techniques such as taking a sexual history, performing a pelvic examination, or doing a surgical procedure.

Discussion moves the learner from a passive to an active role that facilitates the acquisition of new knowledge. Much of the learning that occurs in a discussion format depends on the instructor's skills in creating a supportive learning climate, assessing learners' needs, and effectively using a variety of interventions such as maintaining focus, questioning, generalizing, and summarizing for the learner (7–8). *Group discussion* of cases, as in attending rounds or in morning report, is a popular method that allows learners to process new knowledge with faculty and peers and to identify specific knowledge deficiencies. Group discussions are most successful when teachers trained in the techniques of small-group teaching facilitate those discussions (8–11) and when participants have some background knowledge or experience. Preparatory readings can help. The *combination of lecture and small-group discussion* can be extremely effective in imparting knowledge, as well as in practicing the higher-order cognitive skills of assessment and integration of medical facts. *Individual instruction,* or *one-on-one teaching,* has the ability to be the most learner-centered technique, as well as to require active participation on the part of the learner. However, it is faculty intensive and does not provide opportunity for peer interaction.

Programmed learning (12) refers to the use of programmed textbooks or computers that present material in organized sequential fashion, such as the computer-based patient questions being developed by the National Board of Medical Examiners (NBME). Learners using these systems can proceed at their own pace, identify their own knowledge deficiencies, and set their own objectives, as well as receive immediate feedback, not only on their knowledge base, but also on efficiency and cost-effectiveness. Programmed learning materials are now available for a number of content areas. If not previously developed, the costs of developing such materials may be high.

> **EXAMPLE:** *Syllabus Materials.* To teach medical students how to critically appraise the literature, a curriculum was designed that introduced problem-based educational materials into the weekly clerkship tutorial, including (a) a set of objectives and guidelines for how to use the package, (b) a patient scenario presenting a clinical dilemma, (c) a relevant journal article, and (d) an essay defining and discussing quality standards that should be met by the article. A worksheet was provided for each journal article (13).

> **EXAMPLE:** *Specifically Prepared Readings with Questions and Patient Case Scenarios.* The American College of Physicians' Medical Knowledge Self-Assessment Program consists of annotated syllabi in different internal medicine subspecialties, self-assessment questions, and patient case scenarios. Participants can review the information, self-test at their own pace, and receive feedback on their performance at regular intervals. Regional courses are offered to supplement the program. References are provided for further reading.

> **EXAMPLE:** *Computer-Based Program That Includes Readings, Lectures, and Audiovisual Materials.* A recently published CD-ROM in clinical dermatology presents clinical photographs, diagnostic guides, and treatment regimens by diagnosis. Video segments demonstrate surgical procedures, and audio segments include brief lectures on selected topics (*Clinical Dermatology Illustrated,* through Continuing Medical Education Associates, Inc.).

Methods for Achieving Affective Objectives

Methods that are commonly used to achieve affective objectives include the following:

- Exposure (readings, discussions, experiences)
- Facilitation of openness, introspection, and reflection
- Role models

Attitudes can be difficult to measure, let alone change (14). Some undesirable attitudes are based in insufficient knowledge and will change as knowledge is expanded in a particular area. Other attitudes, expressed, for example, by "This is not my responsibility," may be based in insufficient skill or lack of confidence. Attitudinal change requires *exposure to knowledge, experiences, or the views of respected others that contradict undesired and confirm desired attitudes* (15). Targeted readings may be helpful adjuncts to other methods for developing desirable attitudes. Probably more than any other learning objective, attitudinal change is helped by the use of *facilitation techniques with individuals and with groups that promote openness, introspection, and reflection* (16–18). These facilitation methods can be incorporated into skill-building methods, such as role-plays or simulated patient exercises, where the learner may be encouraged by the group process to explore barriers to performance. Properly facilitated small-group discussions can also promote changes in attitudes by bringing into awareness the interests, attitudes, values, and feelings of learners and by making them available for discussion. Finally, *role model* health professionals can help change attitudes by demonstrating successful approaches to a particular problem. Interestingly, the professional attitudes that educators often aim to instill in students, such as competency, excellence, sensitivity, enthusiasm, and genuineness, are those attributes that students value most in their teachers (19–21).

> **EXAMPLE:** *Attitude toward Role.* A geriatrics curriculum has as an objective that primary care residents will believe it is their role to document advance directive wishes of their elderly outpatients. A needs assessment instrument discovers that most residents believe that their patients do not want these discussions or have no biases about advance directives. A videotape interview of a respected geriatrician with several of his patients is used to model the technique of the advance directive interview as well as the reaction of patients to the discussion. The videotape is used as a trigger tape in small group discussions of residents to discuss the physician's role in and patient reactions to such discussions.

> **EXAMPLE:** *Attitude toward Socioeconomic Class.* A residency program has as a goal that its graduates will be sensitive to sociocultural issues affecting vulnerable patient populations. Two strategies have been introduced into the curriculum. First, block ambulatory residents are required to document an hour interview with a patient whom they know well, to listen to the patient's life history rather than perform a traditional medical interview, and to present the case in the context of economics, nutrition, housing, and the social history of a population. Second, during monthly medical anthropology rounds, cases raising issues of cross-cultural health care are discussed in the presence of a community leader (22).

> **EXAMPLE:** *Awareness and Management of Negative Feelings.* In a substance abuse and HIV curriculum, residents watch a trigger tape of a difficult interaction between a substance-abusing HIV-infected patient and a physician. They identify and discuss the emotions and attitudes evoked by the tape and reflect upon how these feelings might influence their management of such patients. Subsequently, residents work with a highly respected role model physician in a practice that successfully manages such patients.

Methods for Achieving Psychomotor Objectives

Skill or Competency Objectives.   Methods commonly used to achieve skill or competency objectives include the following:

- Supervised clinical experiences
- Simulations
    Artificial models
    Role-Plays
    Standardized patients
- Audio or visual reviews of skills

Rarely is knowledge the sole prerequisite to a learner's achievement of competence in a health-related area. In medicine, learners need to develop a variety of skills, including basic auditory and visual skills of the physical examination, manual skills for procedures and techniques, and communication skills in the medical interview. The learning of skills can be facilitated when learners

a. receive an *introduction* to the skills by didactic presentations, demonstration, and discussion;
b. have the opportunity to *practice* the skills;
c. have the opportunity to *reflect* upon their performance;
d. receive *feedback* on their performance;
e. *repeat the cycle* of discussion, practice, reflection, and feedback until mastery is achieved.

The development of experiential learning methods can be a creative process for curriculum developers, one that provides an opportunity for innovation in medical education. Experiential learning can be challenging for the learner and teacher alike. Experiential learning requires learners to expose their strengths and weaknesses to themselves and others. Interpersonal skills, feelings, biases, psychological defenses, and previous experiences may affect performance and need to be discussed. Creation of a *safe and supportive learning environment* is, therefore, helpful. Methods include the development of faculty-learner rapport, disclosure by faculty of their own experiences and difficulties with the material, explicit recognition and reinforcement of the learner's strengths, and provision of feedback about deficiencies in a factual, nonjudgmental, helpful, and positive manner.

The classic experiential method of medical training is the *see one–do one–teach one* approach that occurs daily in clinical settings. Inherent in the success of this method is modeling of the ideal behavior or skill by an experienced clinician, the availability of clinical opportunities for the learner to practice the skill under observation, time to reflect and receive feedback on performance (23), and, lastly, the opportunity to teach the skill to another generation of learners. Effective clinical teachers can facilitate this type of experience (see General References at end of chapter).

EXAMPLE: *Supervised Clinical Experience.* To train internal medicine residents in adequate performance of the pelvic examination, faculty for an ambulatory gynecology curriculum created a checklist of tasks and behaviors to be executed during the examination, including attention to patient comfort, correct order of examination, and proper technique for the PAP smear. Residents attend a family planning clinic, observe the demonstration of pelvic examination technique by a faculty member, and perform pelvic examinations observed by faculty, after which they receive oral feedback on their performance and written feedback through the checklist instrument. These residents are likely, in the future, to demonstrate the procedure to and supervise some medical students or interns in their performance of pelvic examinations.

When expert clinicians are not readily available for demonstration or when the appropriate clinical situations are not available for practice, supplementary methods should be considered. *Videotapes* can be used to demonstrate a skill before the learner practices in another situation. *Simulations* of clinical situations provide the opportunity for learners to practice skills in a "safe" learning environment where risks can be taken and mistakes made without harm. Simulations include the use of artificial models, role-playing, and standardized (or simulated) patients.

Artificial models are inanimate devices designed to simulate real clinical situations. They are usually used as aids for teaching physical examination skills.

EXAMPLE: *Artificial Models.* Devices that simulate heart sounds for developing cardiac auscultation skills (e.g., the Virtual Heart Model for teaching cardiac physiology and physical diagnosis—http://mchip00.nyu.edu/med-ed/virtual heart); breast models for teaching the breast examination, and pelvic models for teaching pelvic examination and PAP smear techniques.

Role-playing, during which the learner plays one role (e.g., physician) and another learner or faculty member plays another role (e.g., patient), provides the opportunity for learners to experience different roles (24). Role-playing is most useful for teaching interviewing skills, physical examination techniques, and the recognition of normal physical examination findings. It permits the learner to try, observe, and discuss alternative techniques until a satisfactory performance has been achieved. It is efficient, inexpensive, and portable and can be used spontaneously in any setting. Role-plays can be constructed on the spot to address individual learner needs as they are identified. Limitations include variable degrees of artificiality, as well as learner and faculty discomfort with the technique. Students are often uncomfortable with this method initially. Facilitators can alleviate this discomfort by discussing it at the outset, by establishing ground rules for the role-play, and by attending to the creation of a safe and supportive learning environment (see above).

EXAMPLE: *Role-Play, Video Review.* A group of medical school faculty sought additional training in the skills of the medical interview, as part of a faculty development program. Participants were videotaped in a role play of giving bad news to a patient. The participants reflected on their performance, received feedback from the other participants in the role play, and from the group at large, and defined areas for continued improvement.

EXAMPLE: *Ground Rules for Role-Play:* The following ground rules are used for setting up and debriefing role plays:

Preparation
- Choose a situation that is relevant and readily conceptualized by the learners.
- Describe the situation and critical issues for each role-playing participant.
- Choose/assign roles and give learners time to assimilate and add details.
- Identify observers and clarify their functions.
- Establish expectations for time-outs by the learner and for interruptions by others (e.g., time limits).

Execution
- Ensure compliance with agreed-upon ground rules.
- Ensure that learners emerge comfortably from their roles.

Debriefing
- First give the principal learner the opportunity to self-assess what he or she did well, would want to do differently, and would like help with.
- Assess the feelings and experiences of other participants in the role-playing exercise.
- Elicit feedback from all observers on what seemed to go well.
- Elicit suggestions regarding alternative approaches that might have been more effective.

Replay
- Give the principal learner the opportunity to repeat the role-playing exercise using alternative approaches.

Standardized (simulated) patients are actors or real patients trained to play the roles of patients with specific problems. As with role-playing, the use of standardized patients ensures that important content areas will be covered and allows learners to try new techniques, make mistakes, and repeat their performance until a skill is achieved. Standardized patients can be trained to provide feedback and instruction, even in the absence of a faculty member. The method has proven efficacy, both for teaching and for evaluating learners (25, 26). Generally, new learners encounter less artificiality and discomfort with standardized patients than with role-playing. The major limitation is the need to recruit, train, schedule, and pay standardized patients (27).

> **EXAMPLE:** *Use of Standardized Patients in Medical Schools.* In a survey of U.S. medical schools (28), 80% used standardized patients for either teaching or evaluation. Sixty percent used standardized patients to teach medical students the breast and pelvic examination; 55%, interviewing skills; 47%, medical history taking; 43%, the male genitourinary examination; 41%, other segments of the physical examination; 40%, focused encounters; 29%, the complete physical examination; and 28%, patient education and counseling. The length of the teaching encounters averaged about 30 minutes, but varied from 10 minutes to two hours. The predominant format for feedback was immediate verbal feedback provided by the standardized patient and/or faculty. Verbal feedback was often supplemented by the provision of written feedback.

Review of taped (audio or video) performances of role-play, standardized patient, or real-patient encounters can serve as helpful adjuncts to experiential learning (29–31). The tapes can provide information on learner and patient behaviors, which may not have been noticed or remembered by the participants. The tapes provide learners with the rare opportunity to observe their own performance from outside of themselves. Properly facilitated audio or video reviews promote helpful reflection on and discussion of a learner's performance.

Behavioral or Performance Objectives.   Methods commonly used to achieve behavioral or performance objectives include the following:

- Removal of barriers to performance
- Provision of resources that facilitate performance
- Provision of reinforcements for performance

Changing learners' behaviors can be one of the more challenging aspects of a curriculum. There is no guarantee that helping learners develop new skills, and even improved attitudes, will result in the desired performance when learners are in actual clinical situations. Skill training is necessary but not sufficient to ensure performance in real settings. In order to promote desired performance, curriculum developers may need to address *barriers to performance* in the learners' environment, provide *resources that promote performance,* and design *reinforcements* that will encourage the continued use of the newly acquired skills. Attention to the learner's subsequent environment can reduce or eliminate the decay of performance that often occurs after an educational intervention.

> **EXAMPLE:** A curriculum in assessing fall risk was introduced to geriatric fellows after a chart audit indicated a neglect in this area in their geriatric outpatient practice. In addition to lectures and discussions, the curriculum developers placed fall-risk questions on the previsit questionnaire completed by patients and added a trigger question on the problem list face sheets of patients' charts. The assessment of fall risk is included in the annual chart audit, and results are fed back to each fellow.

Methods for Promoting Learner-Centeredness

Methods for promoting learner-centeredness include the following:

- Formal or informal assessment of learner needs
- Tailoring of educational content and methods to meet learners' needs

A curriculum is learner-centered to the extent that it is tailored to meet the specific needs of its individual learners and its targeted group of learners. This could mean a) adapting methods to specific learning styles or preferences; b) addressing specific learner needs in the cognitive, affective, or psychomotor areas related to established curricular objectives; or c) accommodating specific learner objectives not included in the curriculum. The success of the established curriculum will be enhanced to the extent that a curriculum can be learner-centered in the first two ways. A curriculum will be richer and more helpful to individual learners than it otherwise would have been to the extent that it can be learner-centered in the third way without detracting from the overall goals of the curriculum.

The *needs assessment of targeted learners* discussed previously is the first step in tailoring a curriculum to a specific group of learners. *Formal evaluators of individual learners,* such as pretests, and *informal observations of individual learners,* which can occur during small-group and one-on-one teaching sessions, can help faculty identify the needs of individual learners. So can *discussion with individual learners,* during which learners are asked about their learning style preferences and perceived needs. This discovery process is more likely to occur when faculty use observational, listening, and question-asking skills.

Once faculty are aware of these specific needs, they may be able to modify or add to the curriculum's educational strategies in order to address the specific needs. Such accommodation is more likely to be possible in *one-on-one* and *small-group teaching* than in lecture situations.

Generally speaking, learner-centered approaches to education require more time and effort on the part of educators than teacher-centered approaches do. Learner-centered approaches, however, are more likely to engage the learner and succeed in helping the learner achieve agreed-upon objectives. The curriculum developer will need to decide to what extent learner-centered approaches are (a) crucial to the achievement of curricular objectives, (b) desirable but not crucial, and (c) feasible within resource constraints.

EXAMPLE: At the beginning of a rotation in communication skills and the psychosocial domain of medical practice, PGY-1 residents assess their competencies and learning needs. The self-assessments are shared with course faculty. Most of the learning in the course occurs in small-group or one-on-one sessions that employ experiential methods (role-plays, standardized patients, video reviews of actual patient encounters). The faculty use information from the self-assessments and from their own observations of learner performance to tailor their approaches to address individual learner needs (31).

EXAMPLE: Students studying biochemistry receive a set of objectives that outlines both the minimum requirement of the course and those areas that students can study in more depth. Students study the subject individually from printed material or programmed tape/slide presentations at their own pace. They may also choose those materials that best suit their learning styles. When the students feel they have mastered a phase of the course, they arrange for an assessment. If they have not achieved an acceptable level of competency, a remedial program of instruction is developed by the staff and student (32).

Methods for Promoting Self-Directed Learning

These methods (33, 34) include the following:

- Training in skills relevant to self-directed learning
    Self-assessment
    Information searching
    Critical appraisal
    Clinical decision making
- Independent-Learning Projects
- Personal-Learning Plans or Contracts
- Formulating and answering one's own questions
- Role Modeling

In an era of burgeoning information and ever-evolving advances in medical care, it is important for curriculum developers to consider how learners will continue to develop in relevant cognitive, affective, and psychomotor areas after completion of the curriculum. Most overall educational programs have as a stated or unstated goal that their learners, by the end of the program, will be effective self-directed learners. *Effective self-directed learners* take primary responsibility for their own learning, accurately identify their own learning needs, clarify their learning goals and objectives, successfully identify and use resources and educational strategies that can help them achieve their goals and objectives, accurately assess their achievements, and repeat the learning cycle if necessary. By its very nature, self-directed learning is learner-centered. An advantage of self-directed learning is that active learners are said to learn more things more efficiently, to retain that knowledge better, and to use it more effectively than passive learners do (34).

A self-directed learning approach is most applicable when the learner already has some relevant knowledge and experience. It is easiest when the learner already possesses *skills that facilitate self-directed learning* such as self-assessment skills, library and informatics skills for searching the health care literature and other databases, skills in reading and critically appraising the medical literature, and clinical decision-making skills.

Curriculum developers must decide how their curriculum will fit into an educational program's overall approach to promoting the development of self-directed learners. If the curriculum being developed is located toward the beginning of a multifaceted educational program, it may need to take responsibility for teaching learners skills relevant to a self-directed-learning approach (see above). If learners have already developed these fundamental skills, but are relatively inexperienced in self-directed learning, they may benefit from a special orientation to self-directed learning and from an intensive mentoring process. If an effective self-directed-learning approach has already been established in the overall program, the curriculum can simply include methods with which the learners are already familiar.

Required *independent learning projects and reports* are the method that is most commonly used to promote self-directed learning. Curricula can also require that learners develop a *personal learning plan or contract* (35), usually in combination with a preceptor or mentor, that specifies learning objectives, learning methods, resources, and evaluation methods. Faculty can promote self-directed learning by encouraging *targeted independent reading or consultation* related to problems that are encountered, by *encouraging and helping learners to answer some of their own questions,* and by *modeling* self-directed learning themselves.

A curriculum is most likely to be successful in promoting self-directed learning if it schedules sufficient protected time for the activity, clearly communicates expectations to the learner, requires products (e.g., formal or informal presentations or reports), provides ongoing mentoring and supervision throughout the process, and provides training for learners in skills that facilitate self-directed learning if they are lacking.

> **EXAMPLE:** All PGY-1 residents are assigned to a one-month rotation in which they learn informatics, critical appraisal, and clinical decision-making skills. Residents are required to apply these skills by critically assessing a clinical practice of their choice. At the end of the month, they formally present their findings to an invited audience. Time is provided within the curriculum for residents to work on their projects.

Methods for Promoting Teamwork

Methods that can be used to help learners develop as effective team members include the following:

- Collaborative-learning experiences
- Work environments that model effective teamwork
- Assessments of team function
- Training in team skills

As medical knowledge has increased, and as societal expectations for customer-responsive, high-quality, cost-effective care have risen, the mechanisms for providing the best health care have become more complex (36). It is becoming unlikely that an independent practitioner will be able to provide the best care to individual patients, a panel of patients, or the community. Rather, health care professionals will have to work effectively in teams to accomplish desired goals (36–39).

Accordingly, medical curricula that have traditionally fostered a competitive approach to learning, and an autocratic approach to providing care, now need to foster collaborative approaches to learning and to prepare learners to be effective team members. Health care professionals need to become knowledgeable about and skilled in facilitating group process (40), in running and participating in meetings (41), in being appropriately assertive (42), in managing conflict (43), in facilitating organizational change (44), in motivating others (45, 46), in delegating and supervising others (47), and in feedback (23) and general communication skills (48).

Some curricula may be developed to specifically address these skills. Other curricula may focus upon the teamwork skills and behaviors that health care professionals will need to solve the health care problems specific to the curricula. Most curricula should reinforce team skills that are objectives of the overall educational program, of which the curricula are a part. Methods for promoting and reinforcing team skills include fostering collaborative (49) versus competitive approaches to learning, exposing learners to clinical and other experiences that model effective teamwork, arranging for some of the learning to occur in properly facilitated small groups, encouraging or requiring independent projects by small groups as well as by individuals, having learners assess and discuss the functioning of the teams in which they have been involved, and focusing curricula on team functioning and related skills.

EXAMPLE: In a faculty development workshop for curriculum development, groups of two to five faculty work over nine months to develop and pilot medical curricula. At the beginning of the workshop, a facilitator guides participants in a discussion of effective group behaviors and provides participants with a group-process rating sheet by which to evaluate their own groups. With this background, workshop participants throughout the year are asked to reflect on the functioning of their groups and on the effect of group process on their curricular projects.

CONCLUSION

The challenge of Step 4 is to devise educational strategies that achieve the curricular objectives set out in Step 3, within the resource constraints of available time, space, money, clinical material, and faculty. The need to promote learner-centeredness, self-directed learning, and teamwork may be additional considerations that are consistent with initiatives in the overall training program or school or consistent with the educational philosophy of the curriculum developers themselves. Creativity in the development of educational strategies is an opportunity for scholarship, particularly if the curriculum is carefully evaluated, as we shall see in a subsequent chapter.

QUESTIONS

For the curriculum you are coordinating, planning, or would like to be planning please answer the following:

1. In the table below write one important, specific measurable objective in each of the following domains: cognitive, affective, and psychomotor.

2. Choose educational methods from Table 5.3 to achieve each of your educational objectives.

3. Is each educational method congruent with the domain of its objective?

4. Are you concerned that there will be a decay over time in the achievement of any of your objectives?

5. From Tables 5.2 and 5.3, choose an additional method for each objective that would most likely prevent decay after the achievement of the objective.

6. Identify the resources that you will need to implement your educational methods. Consider available teachers in your institution, costs for simulations or clinical experiences, time, and space. Are your methods feasible?

	Domain of the Objective		
	Cognitive (Knowledge)	Affective (Attitude)	Psychomotor (Skill or Performance)
Specific Measurable Objectives			
Educational Method to Achieve			
Educational Method to Prevent Decay			
Resources Required			

7. Have you included any methods that are learner-centered or that promote self-directed learning? If yes, what are they?

8. Will your curriculum include educational strategies that promote effective teamwork? Why or why not? If yes, what are they?

9. Have the methods you suggested in your answers to questions 7 or 8 affected your need for resources? How? Are your methods feasible?

GENERAL REFERENCES

General References on learning, instructional design, and teaching are included here. References on specific educational/teaching methods are included under the Specific References section and are cited in the text.

American College of Physicians Governors' Class of 1996. *Learning from Practitioners: Office-Based Teaching of Internal Medicine.* Philadelphia: American College of Physicians; 1995.
   This work, written by medical practitioners, is a practical, useful manual on teaching in ambulatory, office-based (as opposed to hospital-based) settings. 40 pages.

Cross KP. *Adults as Learners.* San Francisco: Jossey-Bass; 1988.
   Written for educators and trainers of adult learners in any discipline or profession, the book describes and synthesizes research findings into two explanatory models: one for understanding motivations of adult learners and the other for organizing knowledge about the characteristics of adult learners. There is also a chapter on facilitation. 300 pages.

Davis DA, Fox RD, eds. *The Physician as Learner: Linking Research to Practice.* Chicago: American Medical Association, 1994.
This multiauthored, but reader-friendly, text focuses on the physician as learner, on assessment of learning needs, and on continuing medical education [CME]. 366 pages.

Dick W, Carey L. *The Systematic Design of Instruction.* 3d ed. Glenview, Ill.: Scott, Foresman; 1990.
The authors present a framework for instructional design very similar to that proposed in this chapter. The book places particular emphasis on behavioral objectives, preinstructional activities, student participation, and testing. Chapters 8 and 9 address the development of instructional strategy and selection of instructional materials. Specific (non-health-related) examples are detailed in the text. 351 pages.

Douglas KC, Hosokawa MC, Lawler FH. *A Practical Guide to Clinical Teaching in Medicine.* New York: Springer Publishing; 1988.
One of a series on medical education, this book is a succinct and readable guide to clinical teaching, with a brief background in adult learning theory and with helpful hints for implementing curricula. Chapters 8 and 9 address strategies for learning in the cognitive, affective, and psychomotor domains. 191 pages.

Ende J, Atkins E. Conceptualizing curriculum for graduate medical education. *Acad Med* 1992; 67:528–534.
This article discusses limitations of objectives-driven curricula and how to structure educational programs to maximize learning from experience. (See also discussion at end of Chapter 4, Step 4: Goals and Objectives.)

Green LW, Kreuter MW, Deeds SG, Partridge KB. Selection of educational strategies. In *Health Education Planning: A Diagnostic Approach.* Palo Alto, Calif.: Mayfield Publishing; 1980. Pp. 86–115.
This classic text uses a conceptual framework for planning and implementing health programs. The framework includes epidemiologic diagnosis/health problem definition, behavioral and educational diagnosis, social/community/target group factors, and administrative diagnosis. Chapter 6 discusses the selection of educational strategies in the context of this framework. The book is oriented to educational interventions for communities and patient populations, but the concepts are also applicable to educational programs targeted at health professionals. 306 pages.

Harden RM, Sowden S, Dunn WR. Education strategies in curriculum development: The SPICES model. *Med Educ* 1984; 18:284–297.
This paper provides a concise summary of six strategies in medical education which are represented as a continuum of dichotomous approaches: (1) student (learner)-centered/teacher-centered; (2) problem-based/information-gathering; (3) integrated/discipline-based; (4) community-based/hospital-based; (5) elective/uniform program; and (6) systematic/apprenticeship-opportunistic. Each approach is defined, and its strengths and weaknesses noted. The paper provides another set of criteria by which to classify curricular strategies.

Romiszowski AJ. *Designing Instructional Systems: Decision Making in Course Planning and Curriculum Design.* New York: Nichols Publishing; 1981.
This book proposes a model of instructional macrodesign, based on four levels: theories and philosophies, instructional strategies, instructional plans, and instructional tactics. 415 pages.

Romiszowski AJ. *Producing Instructional Systems: Lesson Planning for Individualized and Group Learning Activities.* New York: Nichols Publishing; 1984.
This book provides a focus on microdesign or instructional tactics: lesson planning for individualized instruction in a classroom environment, as well as planning of small-group learning situations, simulations, and games. 286 pages.

Romiszowski, AJ. *The Selection and Use of Instructional Media for Improved Classroom Teaching and for Interactive, Individualized Instruction.* 2d ed. New York: Nichols Publishing, 1988.
This book presents a detailed approach to the use of instructional media, from printed word to interactive networking. 396 pages.

Rubenstein W, Talbot Y. *Medical Teaching in Ambulatory Care: A Practical Guide.* New York: Springer Publishing; 1992.
    This is a short, practical, useful text on office-based precepting that includes a section on challenging learning situations. 126 pages.

Schwenk TL, Whitman NA. *The Physician as Teacher.* Baltimore: Williams and Wilkins; 1987.
    This book discusses teaching as a form of communication and relationship; it also discusses specific teaching responsibilities: lectures, group discussions, teaching rounds and morning report, bedside teaching, and teaching in the ambulatory setting. 203 pages.

Whitman NA, Schwenk TL. *Preceptors as Teachers: A Guide to Clinical Teaching.* Salt Lake City: University of Utah School of Medicine; 1984.
    This is an excellent, practical, pithy text that covers the essentials of clinical teaching. 25 pages.

Whitman NA. *Creative Medical Teaching.* Salt Lake City: University of Utah, School of Medicine; 1990.
    This book conveys wisdom and information in a readable format with a detailed table of contents permitting selective reading of educational principles, methods, and examples. 232 pages.

SPECIFIC REFERENCES

1. Price GE. Diagnosing learning styles. In Smith RM, *Helping Adults Learn How to Learn.* San Francisco: Jossey-Bass, 1983. Pp. 49–55.
2. Hilliard RI. How do medical students learn? Medical student learning styles and factors that affect these learning styles. *Teaching and Learning in Medicine* 1995; 7:201–210.
3. Fairman RP, Robichaud AM, Glauser FL. Is anyone out there listening? The art and science of lecturing. *Medical Times* 1989; 117:124–130.
4. Schwenk TL, Whitman NA. Lectures. In Schwenk TL, Whitman NA, eds., *The Physician as Teacher.* Baltimore: Williams and Wilkins; 1987. Pp. 71–90.
5. Westberg J, Jason H. *Making Presentations: A Guide Book for Health Professions Teachers.* Boulder, Colo.: Center for Instructional Support; 1991. Pp. 1–89.
6. Whitman NA. *There Is No Gene for Good Teaching: A Handbook on Lecturing for Medical Teachers.* Salt Lake City: University of Utah School of Medicine; 1982.
7. Knowles MS. *Self-Directed Learning: A Guide for Learners and Teachers.* New York: Cambridge (The Adult Education Co.); 1975. Pp. 9–11, 29–38, 99–103.
8. Whitman NE, Schwenk TL. *A Handbook for Group Discussion Leaders: Alternatives to Lecturing Medical Students to Death.* Salt Lake City: University of Utah School of Medicine; 1983. Pp. 1–38.
9. Schwenk TL, Whitman NA. Group discussions. In Schwenk TL, Whitman NA, eds., *The Physician as Teacher.* Baltimore: Williams and Wilkins; 1987 pp. 91–100.
10. Tiberius RG. *Small-Group Teaching: A Trouble-Shooting Guide.* Toronto: Ontario Institute for Studies in Education Press; 1990. Pp. 1–194.
11. Westburg J, Jason H. *Fostering Learning in Small Groups: A Practical Guide.* New York: Springer Publishing; 1996. Pp. 1–267.
12. Romiszowski AJ. *Developing Auto-instructional Materials: From Programmed Texts to CAL and Interactive Video.* New York: Nichols Publishing; 1986. Pp. 131–153, 298–304.
13. Bennett CJ, Sackett DL, Haynes RB, Neufeld VR, Tugwell P. Roberts R. A controlled trial of teaching critical appraisal of the clinical literature to medical students. *JAMA* 1987; 257:2451–2454.
14. Henerson ME, Morris LL, Fitz-Gibbon CT. *How to Measure Attitudes* (book number 6). In *Program Evaluation Kit.* Newbury Park, Calif.: Sage Publications; 1987. Pp. 9–13.

15. Dick W, Carey L. *The Systematic Design of Instruction.* 3d ed. Glenview, Ill.: Scott, Foresman; 1990. Pp. 171–173.
16. Bentley TJ. *Facilitation: Providing Opportunities for Learning.* Berkshire, England: McGraw-Hill; 1994. Pp. 25–60.
17. Brookfield SD. *Understanding and Facilitating Adult Learning.* San Francisco: Jossey-Bass; 1987. Pp. 123–126.
18. Rogers CR. Significant learning in therapy and education. In Rogers CR, *On Becoming a Person: A Therapist's View of Psychology.* Boston: Houghton Mifflin, 1961. Pp. 279–296.
19. Whitman NA, Schwenk TL. *Preceptors as Teachers: A Guide to Clinical Teaching.* Salt Lake City: University of Utah School of Medicine; 1982. P. 17.
20. Wright S, Wong A, Newill C. The impact of role models on medical students. *J Gen Intern Med* 1997; 12:53–56.
21. Wright S. Examining what residents look for in their role models. *Acad Med* 1996; 71:290–292.
22. Lurie N, Yergan J. Teaching residents to care for vulnerable populations in the outpatient setting. *J Gen Intern Med* 1990; 5(suppl.):S27–S34.
23. Ende J. Feedback in clinical medical education. *JAMA* 1983; 250(6):777–781.
24. Simpson MA. How to use role-play in medical teaching. *Medical Teacher* 1985; 7:75–82.
25. Stillman PL, Swanson D, Regan B et al. Assessment of clinical skills of residents utilizing standardized patients. *Ann Intern Med* 1991; 114:393–401.
26. Stillman PL, Burpeau-DeGaegorio MY, Nicholson GI, Sabers DL, Stillman AE. Six years of experience using patient instructors to teach interviewing skills. *J Med Educ* 1983; 58:941–946.
27. King AM, Perkowski-Roberts LC, Pohl HS. Planning standardized patient programs: case development, patient training, and costs. *Teaching and Learning in Medicine* 1994; 6:6–14.
28. Anderson MB, Stillman PL, Wang Y. Growing use of standardized patients in teaching and evaluation in medical education. *Teaching and Learning in Medicine* 1994; 6:15–22.
29. Edwards A, Tzelepis A, Klingbeil C et al. Fifteen years of a videotape review program for internal medicine and medicine-pediatrics residents. *Acad Med* 1996; 71:744–748.
30. Scheidt PC, Lazoritz S, Ebbeling WE, Figelman HR, Moessner HF, Singer JE. Evaluation of a system providing feedback on videotaped patient encounters. *J Med Educ* 1986; 61:585–590.
31. Kern DE, Grayson M, Barker LR, Roca RP, Cole KA, Roter D, Golden AS. Residency training in interviewing skills and the psychosocial domain of medical practice. *J Gen Intern Med* 1989; 4:421–431.
32. Harden RM, Snowden S, Dunn WR. Educational strategies in curriculum development: The SPICES model. *Med Educ* 1984; 18:284–297.
33. Brookfield S. ed. *Self-Directed Learning: From Theory to Practice.* San Francisco: Jossey-Bass; 1985.
34. Knowles MS. *Self-Directed Learning: A Guide for Learners and Teachers.* New York: Cambridge (The Adult Education Co.); 1975.
35. Knowles MS. *Using Learning Contracts.* San Francisco: Jossey-Bass; 1986.
36. Pew Health Professions Commission. Health professions education and managed care: Challenges and necessary responses. Report, August 1995. Pp. 9–20.
37. Manion J, Lorimer W, Leander WJ. *Team-Based Health Care Organizations: Blueprint for Success.* Gaithersburg, Md.: Aspen Publications; 1996.
38. Pritchard P, Pritchard J. *Developing Teamwork in Primary Health Care: A Practical Workbook.* Oxford, England: Oxford University Press; 1992.
39. Quick TL. *Successful Team Building.* New York: American Management Association; 1992.
40. Westberg J, Jason H. Facilitating discussions and dialogues. In *Fostering Learning in Small Groups: A Practical Guide.* New York: Springer Publishing; 1996. Pp. 127–155.
41. Doyle M, Straus D. *How to Make Meetings Work.* New York: Berkley Publishing Group; 1982. Pp. 1–298.
42. Lange AJ, Jakubowski P. *Responsible Assertive Behavior: Cognitive/Behavioral Procedures for Trainers.* Champaign, Ill.: Research Press; 1976. Pp. 7–53.

43. Fisher R, Ury W. *Getting to Yes.* New York: Penguin; 1981. Pp. 1–200.

44. Depree M. *Leadership Is an Art.* New York: Dell Publishing; 1989. Pp. 31–43.

45. Byham WC. *Zapp! The Lightning of Empowerment.* New York: Fawcett Columbine; 1988. Pp. 3–191.

46. Byham WC. *Zapp! Empowerment in Health Care.* New York: Fawcett Columbine; 1993. Pp. 3–309.

47. Blanchard K, Johnson S. *The One Minute Manager.* New York: Berkley Books; 1983. Pp. 11–111.

48. Timm PR, Stead JA. *Communication Skills for Business and Professions.* Upper Saddle River, N.J.: Prentice Hall; 1996. Pp. 80–97, 112–129.

49. Weinholtz D, Edwards J, Mumford LM. *Teaching during Rounds: A Handbook for Attending Physicians and Residents.* Baltimore: Johns Hopkins University Press; 1992. Pp. 2, 3, 98–100.

CHAPTER SIX

Step 5: Implementation

IMPORTANCE

For a curriculum to achieve its potential, careful attention must be paid to issues of implementation. The curriculum developer must ensure that sufficient resources, political and financial support, and administrative strategies have been developed to successfully implement the curriculum (Table 6.1).

IDENTIFICATION OF RESOURCES

The curriculum developer must realistically assess the resources that will be required to implement the educational strategies (Chapter 5) and the evaluation (Chapter 7) planned for the curriculum. Resources include personnel, time, facilities, and funding.

Table 6.1.   Checklist for Implementation

___ Identify resources
    ___ Personnel: faculty, secretarial and other support staff, patients, other
    ___ Time: faculty, support staff, learners
    ___ Facilities: space, equipment, clinical sites
    ___ Funding/Costs: direct financial costs, hidden or opportunity costs

___ Obtain support
    ___ Internal
            From: those with administrative authority (dean's office, hospital administra-
                tion, department chair, program director, division director, etc.), faculty,
                learners, other stakeholders
            For: personnel, resources, political support
    ___ External
            From: government, professional societies, philanthropic organizations or foun-
                dations, other entities (e.g., managed care organizations), individual donors
            For: funding, political support, curricular or faculty development resources

___ Develop administrative mechanisms to support the curriculum.
    ___ Administrative structure: to delineate responsibilities and decision making
    ___ Communication
            Content: rationale; goals and objectives; information about the curriculum,
                learners, faculty, facilities and equipment, scheduling; changes in the cur-
                riculum; evaluation results; etc.
            Mechanisms: memos, meetings, syllabus materials, site visits, reports, etc.
    ___ Operations: preparation and distribution of schedules and curricular materials;
            collection, collation, and distribution of evaluation data; curricular revisions and
            changes, etc.

___ Anticipate and address barriers.
    ___ Financial and other resources
    ___ Competing demands
    ___ People: attitudes, job/role security, power and authority, etc.

___ Plan to introduce the curriculum.
    ___ Pilot
    ___ Phase-In
    ___ Full Implementation

Personnel

Personnel includes faculty and support staff. Ideally *faculty* will be available and skilled in both teaching and content. If there are insufficient numbers of skilled faculty, one must contemplate hiring new faculty or developing existing faculty.

> **EXAMPLE:** *Faculty Development before the Start of a Curriculum.* A curriculum was devel-
> oped with small-group learning as its main educational method. The faculty was relatively in-
> experienced in this method of teaching. A targeted two-session faculty development program
> on small-group facilitation techniques, and periodic faculty meetings, were held to promote
> faculty acquisition, discussion, and continued development of these skills.

EXAMPLE: *Faculty Development in Response to Evaluation.* Evaluations from an existing clinical skills course for second-year medical students revealed some deficiencies in preceptors' provision of feedback. The course director asked other faculty from the same institution, who were experts in faculty development, to develop a two-and-a-half-hour workshop on feedback skills that could be integrated into the orientation session for course preceptors. After two years of workshops, evaluations reflected an improved performance in this area.

Secretarial and other support staff are usually needed to type curricular materials, prepare and communicate schedules, collect evaluation data, prepare evaluation reports, and support learning activities. Sometimes *additional personnel,* such as standardized patients, will be required. A suitable mix of real *patients* is a "personnel" need that may be necessary to provide learners with crucial clinical experience and should not be overlooked.

Time

Faculty require time to prepare and to teach, as well as time to plan and administer the curriculum. Learners require time not only to attend scheduled learning activities, but to read, reflect, do independent learning, and apply what they have learned. Support staff need time to perform their functions.

Facilities

Curricula require facilities, such as space and equipment. The simplest curriculum may require only a room in which to meet or lecture. Another curriculum may need special equipment, such as audio or video equipment, computers, or artificial models to teach clinical skills. A clinical site that can accommodate learners and provide the appropriate volume and mix of clinical experience may be crucial to yet another curriculum.

Funding/Costs

Sometimes curricula can be accomplished by redeploying existing resources. If this appears to be the case, one should ask what will be given up in redeploying the resources, that is, what is the hidden or opportunity cost of the curriculum? When additional resources are required, they must be provided from somewhere. If additional funding is requested, it is necessary to develop and justify a budget. Whether or not additional funding is requested, it is often useful to determine how a curriculum is funded and what it really costs.

EXAMPLE: For the women's health/gynecology curriculum for general internal medicine (GIM) residents described in examples in Chapters 3, 4, and 5, the following resources were felt necessary: curricular time scheduled into one ambulatory block rotation of each PGY-2 resident; three to four faculty to take responsibility for the didactic sessions; a pelvic model for demonstrating and practicing pelvic examinations and the proper technique for cervical cancer screening; clinical experience with an on-site preceptor, including the appropriate case mix, space, equipment (including examination tables designed for pelvic examinations), and nursing staff; after the curriculum, a continuing clinical experience that provides an opportunity to apply priority skills and management strategies; and a nurse auditor to audit continuity clinic charts with respect to the appropriate provision of cervical cancer screening.

Based upon a needs assessment of GIM residents, the curriculum had been solicited by the GIM division director and GIM residency program director. The division committed a modest amount of funds for salary support of the gynecologist on the original curriculum development team. The time of other GIM and gynecology faculty and fellows, funds for equipment, and curricular time were allocated based upon negotiations between the departments of Medicine and Gynecology, demonstration of the needs of the curriculum, and consideration of other competing needs for a limited pool of resources. The limited nature of the resources helped the curriculum developers to focus their objectives, educational strategies, and requests for resources.

OBTAINING SUPPORT FOR THE CURRICULUM

A curriculum is more likely to be successful in achieving its goals and objectives if it has broad support.

Internal Support

It is important that curriculum developers and coordinators recognize who the stakeholders in a curriculum are, and foster their support. Stakeholders are those individuals who directly affect or are directly affected by a curriculum. For most curricula, stakeholders include individuals with administrative power within the institution, faculty, and learners.

Those with administrative authority (e.g., dean, hospital administrators, department chair, program director, division director) can allocate or deny the funds, space, faculty time, curricular time, and political support that are crucial to a curriculum. *Curricular faculty* can devote varying amounts of their time, enthusiasm, and energy to the curriculum. *Other faculty* who have administrative influence or who may be competitors for curricular space or time can facilitate or create barriers for a curriculum. *Learners'* opinions can influence those with administrative power.

Individuals who feel that a curriculum is important, effective, and popular, who believe that a curriculum positively affects them or their institution, and who have had input into that curriculum are more likely to support it. It is, therefore, helpful to provide stakeholders with the appropriate amount of rationale and evaluation data to address their concerns, and it is helpful to elicit the input of stakeholders as the curriculum is being planned.

> **EXAMPLE:** Evaluations and example videotapes from a curriculum in interviewing skills and the psychosocial domain of medical practice (1), which was developed in 1979 for general internal medicine residents, were shared with the department chairman. As a result the curriculum was expanded in 1983 to include traditional track as well as primary care track residents. When the primary care track lost its federal funding in 1987, consideration was given to eliminating the one-month med-psych rotation. Resident support for the training helped to maintain the curriculum and its associated faculty.

> **EXAMPLE:** An evidence based medicine curriculum was developed in the above primary care track with new federal funding in 1993. It was so popular with the residents and so consistent with the values of internal medicine and the goals of the overall training program that the department chair asked that it be expanded during its second year to include all residents. To accommodate the curriculum, he created a second ambulatory block rotation without inpatient service requirements for the traditional track residents.

External Support

Sometimes there are insufficient institutional resources to support part or all of a curriculum, or to support its further development or expansion. In these situations, a source of external support is critical.

Potential sources of *external funding* (see Appendix B: Additional Resources) include government agencies, professional societies, philanthropic organizations or foundations, other entities (e.g., managed care organizations), and individual donors. Research and development grants may be available from one's own institution, and the competition may be less intense than for truly external funds. External funds are more likely to be obtained when there has been a request for proposals by a funding source, when support is requested for an innovative or particularly needed curriculum, and when the funding is legitimately not available from internal sources. Funding for student summer jobs (usually by universities, professional schools, or professional societies) is another resource that may be available to curricular or evaluation activities in need of support. A period of external funding can be used to build a level of internal support that may sustain the curriculum after cessation of external funding.

> **EXAMPLE:** Federal funding was obtained in 1978 to develop a primary care track within an existing traditional internal medicine training program. From 1978 to 1987, a program was developed that included a much-expanded ambulatory primary care experience, training in interviewing skills and the psychosocial domain of medical practice (med-psych), and ambulatory training in a number of non-internal-medicine specialties. Grant requirements and the provision of funding led to initial political acceptance of these program components by the internal stakeholders. Additional residents were hired to decrease inpatient service requirements, new faculty were hired to teach the med-psych curriculum, and existing GIM faculty increased their administrative and teaching time. The GIM track became a recruiting tool for the residency and developed national recognition and internal support independent of the external support. When federal funding ended in 1987, the hospital funded the additional residency positions, and the physician group funded the additional faculty expenses.

Government, professional societies, and other entities may have *influence,* through their political or funding power, that can affect the degree of internal support for a curriculum. The curriculum developer may want to bring the guidelines or requirements of such bodies to the attention of stakeholders within his or her own institution.

> **EXAMPLE:** ACGME (Accreditation Council for Graduate Medical Education) requirements (2) can have a major influence on a curriculum developer's institution. For example, changing requirements for ambulatory training have resulted in an increased amount of ambulatory training within many residency programs and an increasing demand for high-quality ambulatory training experiences. ACGME requirements for written curricula have resulted in support by many institutions for the development of curricula.

Finally, professional societies or other institutions may have *curricular or facutly development resources* that can be used by curriculum developers.

> **EXAMPLE:** *Curricular Resources.* The American College of Physicians has developed resources (3) and publications (4, 5) that assist in the development of ambulatory and community-based learning in internal medicine for medal students and residents.

> **EXAMPLES:** *Faculty Development Resources.* The Stanford Faculty Development Program (6, 7) offers one month of intensive training in the principles and skills of clinical teaching, the

teaching of preventive medicine, or the teaching of medical decision making, for selected faculty members, who are trained to conduct seminars in these areas for faculty colleagues at their home institutions. The Harvard Macy Institute offers a 19-day program for physician-educators (divided into an 11-day winter and an 8-day spring session). It addresses four major content areas: learning and teaching; curriculum; evaluation; and leadership. The Johns Hopkins Faculty Development Program for Clinician-Educators has developed a consulting service that presents workshops at and works collaboratively with client institutions to help them develop site-specific faculty development activities. McMasters University offers a faculty development course for teachers of evidence-based medicine. The American Academy on Physician and Patient offers one-half-week regional and one-week national faculty development courses for teachers of interviewing skills and the psychosocial domain of medical practice (see Appendix B: Additional Resources).

ADMINISTRATION OF THE CURRICULUM

Administrative Structure

A curriculum does not operate by itself. It requires an administrative structure to assume responsibility, to maintain communication, and to make operational and policy decisions (e.g., Who should one talk to about a problem with the curriculum? When should syllabus material be distributed? When and where will evaluation data be collected? Should there be a midpoint change in curricular content? Should a learner be assigned to a different faculty member?). Often these functions are those of the curriculum coordinator. Some types of decisions can be delegated to the coordinators for subsegments of the curriculum. Major policy changes may best be made with the help of a core faculty group or after even broader input. In any case, a structure for efficient communication and decision making should be established and made clear to faculty, learners, and support staff.

Communication

As implied above, the rationale, goals, and objectives of the curriculum, evaluation results, and changes in the curriculum need to be communicated in appropriate detail to all involved stakeholders. Lines of communication need to be open to and from the stakeholders. Therefore, the curriculum coordinator needs to establish *mechanisms for communication,* such as periodic meetings, memos, syllabi, presentations, site visits or observations, and a policy regarding one's accessibility.

Operations

Finally, *mechanisms need to be developed to ensure that important functions that support the curriculum are performed.* Such functions include preparing and distributing schedules and curricular materials, collecting and collating evaluation data, and supporting the communication function of the curriculum coordinator. Large curricula usually have support staff who can be delegated these functions and who need to be supervised in their performance.

EXAMPLE: The med-psych curriculum described above is coordinated by a behavioral scientist, who is responsible for the scheduling of faculty and residents; distributing syllabus materials; distributing, collecting, and collating evaluation materials; making operational decisions;

and organizing periodic faculty meetings where experiences are shared and revisions made in the curriculum. A division secretary is assigned to provide support to the med-psych coordinator and is responsible for the majority of the work related to scheduling and the distribution and collection of curricular and evaluation materials. The division's evaluation coordinator collates and distributes end-of-year evaluation reports under the supervision of the med-psych coordinator. The med-psych coordinator makes day-to-day operational decisions but uses a core faculty group and sometimes the entire faculty for major policy decisions or curricular revisions.

ANTICIPATING BARRIERS

Before initiating a new curriculum or making changes in an old curriculum, it is helpful to anticipate and address any barriers to their accomplishment. Barriers can relate to finances, other resources, or people (8, 9) (e.g., competing demands for resources; nonsupportive attitudes; issues of job or role security, credit, and political power).

EXAMPLE: *Competition.* In planning the ambulatory component of the internal medicine clerkship for third-year medical students, the curriculum developer anticipated resistance from the inpatient coordinator for the clerkship, based upon loss of curricular time and responsibility/power. The curriculum developer built a well-reasoned argument for the ambulatory component based upon external recommendations and current needs. She ensured student support for the change and ensured the support of crucial faculty. She gained support from the dean's office and was granted additional curricular time for the ambulatory component, which addressed some of the inpatient coordinator's concerns about loss of curricular time for training on the inpatient services. She invited the inpatient coordinator to be on the planning committee for the ambulatory component, to increase his understanding of needs, to promote his sense of ownership and responsibility for the ambulatory component, and to promote coordination of learning and educational methodology between the inpatient and ambulatory components.

EXAMPLE: *Resistance.* The curriculum coordinators for an interviewing skills curriculum anticipated resistance from some residents to the important educational method of role-playing. They opened the first session by exploring residents' previous experiences with role-playing, some positive and some negative. They explored the reasons for the positive and negative experiences as well as the advantages and limitations of role-playing as a learning method. After the discussion, they elicited the residents' commitment to try role-playing. Finally, they established agreed-upon ground rules for the role-plays, and created a positive, helpful, noncritical environment for learning related to the role-plays (see Chapter 5).

INTRODUCING THE CURRICULUM

Piloting

It is important to pilot test crucial segments of a new curriculum on friendly or convenient audiences before formally introducing it. Crucial segments might include needs assessment and evaluation instruments as well as educational methods. Piloting enables curriculum developers to receive critical feedback and to make important revisions that increase the likelihood of successful implementation.

Phasing-In

Phasing-in a complex curriculum, one part at a time or all at once on a subsegment of the targeted learners, permits a focusing of initial efforts, as faculty and staff learn new procedures. When the curriculum represents a cultural shift in an institution or requires attitudinal changes in the stakeholders, introducing the curriculum one step at a time, rather than all at once, can lessen resistance and increase acceptance, particularly if the stakeholders are involved in the process. Like piloting, phasing-in affords the opportunity to have a cycle of experience, feedback, evaluation, and response before full implementation.

Both the piloting and phasing-in approaches to implementing a curriculum advertise it as a curriculum in development, increase participant tolerance and desire to help, decrease faculty resistance to negative feedback, and increase the chance for success of full implementation.

Full Implementation

In general, full implementation should follow a piloting and/or phasing-in experience. Sometimes, however, the demand for a full curriculum for all learners is so pressing, or a curriculum is so limited in scope, that immediate full implementation is preferable. In this case, the first cycle of the curriculum can be considered as a "pilot" cycle, and the evaluation step can be used to provide information that will guide improvements in the next cycle. Of course, a successful curriculum should always be in a stage of continuous improvement as described in Chapter 8.

> **EXAMPLE:** *Pilot and Phase-In.* The needs assessment instrument, evaluation instruments, and selected curricular materials and segments of the women's health/gynecology curriculum described above were initially piloted on other members of the group that was developing the curriculum, then upon selected other faculty, fellows, and residents, including individuals with expertise in curriculum development. Because the curriculum is integrated into residents' ambulatory block rotations and is taught to only a few residents at a time, there was a natural phasing-in experience. These piloting and phasing-in experiences permitted the needs assessment instrument, evaluation instruments, and curricular components to be fine-tuned before full implementation.

> **EXAMPLE:** *Prolonged Phase-In.* When the previously described med-psych curriculum was first introduced in 1979, interviewing skills and the psychosocial domain of medical practice was not a widely accepted part of internal medicine training. It was required and funded, however, by the primary care training grant that the department had received. During the first few years, sessions of the curriculum were cotaught by behavioral science faculty experienced in the teaching of communication skills and psychiatry but not in the practice of internal medicine and by internal medicine faculty interested but inexperienced in teaching the content of the curriculum. The learners were residents who had been recruited specifically for the primary care track and who were generally receptive to the material. The program evolved, based upon development of both the behavioral science and internal medicine faculty, feedback from an interested group of residents, and frequent faculty interaction and observation of residents. Early feedback from residents, for example, led to the abandonment of lectures on interviewing skills and to an increase in the number of sessions devoted to role-playing, simulated patient exercises, and videotape reviews. By 1983, the curriculum was considered so successful that the department contributed additional resources to expand it to include all residents. This is an example of a prolonged phasing-in period that permitted not only time for

revisions in the curriculum but also time for faculty development and some cultural shifts in the internal medicine department.

INTERACTION WITH OTHER STEPS

As one thinks through what is required to implement a curriculum as it has initially been conceived, one often discovers that there are insufficient resources and administrative structures to support such a curriculum. Further prioritization and focusing of curricular objectives, educational strategies, and/or evaluation are then required. For this reason it is usually wise to be thinking of Step 5 (implementation) in conjunction with Step 3 (goals and objectives), Step 4 (educational strategies), and Step 6 (evaluation). Implementation is the step that converts a mental exercise to reality.

QUESTIONS

For the curriculum you are coordinating, planning, or would like to be planning, please answer or think about the questions below. If your thoughts about a curriculum are just beginning, you may wish to answer these questions in the context of a few educational strategies, such as the ones you identified in your answers to the questions at the end of the Chapter 5.

1. What *resources* are required for the curriculum you envision, in terms of personnel, time, and facilities? Did you remember to think of patients as well as faculty and support staff? What are the internal costs of this curriculum? Is there a need for external resources or funding? If there is a need for external funding, construct a budget. Finally, are your curricular plans feasible in terms of the required resources?

2. What is the degree of *support* within your institution for the curriculum? Where will the resistance come from? How could you increase support and decrease resistance? How likely is it that you will get the support necessary? Will external support be necessary? If so, what are possible sources? and what is the nature of the support that is required (e.g., funds, resource materials, political support)?

3. What sort of *administration,* in terms of *administrative structure, communications, and operations,* is necessary to implement and maintain the curriculum? Think of how decisions will be made, how communication will take place, and what operations are necessary for the smooth functioning of the curriculum (e.g., preparation and distribution of schedules, curricular and evaluation materials, evaluation reports).

4. What *barriers* do you anticipate to implementing the curriculum? Develop plans for addressing them.

5. Develop plans to *introduce* the curriculum. What are the most crucial segments of the curriculum that would be a priority for *piloting*? On whom would you pilot it? Can the curriculum be *phased-in* or must it be implemented all at once on all learners? How will you learn from piloting and phasing-in the curriculum? How will you apply this learning to the curriculum?

6. Given your answers to Questions 1 through 5, is your curriculum likely to be feasible and successful? Do you need to go back to the drawing board and alter your approach to some of the steps? Don't be discouraged. It is better to anticipate problems than to discover them too late. Remember, curriculum development is an interactive cyclical process, and each step affects others.

GENERAL REFERENCES

Goodman RM, Steckler AB. Mobilizing organizations for health enhancement: Theories of organizational change. In Glanz K, Lewis FM, Rimer BK, eds., *Health Behavior and Health Education: Theory, Research and Practice.* San Francisco: Jossey-Bass; 1990. Pp. 314–41.
  Implementing new curricula often involves some degree of organizational change. In this book, the history and characteristics of modern organizational development theory are presented with several health and hospital examples.

King JA, Morris LY, Fitz-Gibbon CT. *How to Assess Program Implementation.* Newbury Park, Calif.: Sage Publications; 1987.
  The focus of this book is on planning and executing an evaluation of how well a program has been implemented. Especially useful is the appendix, which contains over 300 questions to consider when evaluating the implementation of a program. The same questions are important to consider when initially planning and implementing a program. 143 pages.

Kolbe LJ, Iverson DC. Implementing comprehensive school health education: Educational innovation and social change. *Health Education Quarterly* 1981; 8:57–80.
  This is a well-written article about school health education programs, with high applicability to curricula in the medical school and hospital teaching environments. Included are sections on five approaches to analyzing program implementation, characteristics of programs that influence their diffusion, four approaches to implementing educational innovations, four levels or stages of implementation, and a section on maintenance or continuation of a health program.

Lemon M, Greer T, Seigel B. Implementation issues in generalist education. *J Gen Intern Med* 1994; 9 (suppl. 1):S98–S104.
  This article states that the implementation of a new generalist program should be planned for in developmental stages: leadership must establish the need for change; curriculum and site issues must be well thought out; program directors must respond to the major concern of community sites, namely, how to minimize disruption of patient care; and ongoing financial support and procedures for evaluation need to be established.

Rogers EM. *Diffusion of Innovations.* New York: Free Press; 1983.
  This classic text describes all aspects and stages of the process whereby new phenomena are adopted and diffused throughout social systems. The book contains a discussion of the elements of diffusion, the history of diffusion research, the innovation-development process, the innovation-decision process, attributes of innovations and their rate of adoption, opinion leadership and diffusion networks, innovations in organizations, and consequences of innovations. Education, public health, and medical sociology, among other disciplines, have made practical use of the theory and empirical research of Rogers's work. The specific section on implementation [pp. 174–175] is brief but highlights the great importance of implementation to the diffusion process. 453 pages.

Romiszowski AJ. Why projects fail. Chapter 30 in *Designing Instructional Systems: Decision Making in Course Planning and Curriculum Design.* New York: Nichols Publishing; 1981.
  This chapter details the stages of implementing an educational program, sources of potential failure in those stages, and how to avoid failure in those stages.

Scheirer MA, Shediac MC, Cassady CE. Measuring the implementation of health promotion programs: the case of the Breast and Cervical Cancer Program in Maryland. *Health Education Research* 1995; 10(1):11–25.

> This paper addresses the important issues and benefits of measuring the extent and processes of program implementation when conducting health education programs. The content is easily transferable to the importance of implementation in medical education programs.

Whitman N, Weiss E, Bishop FM, eds. *Executive Skills for Medical Faculty.* Salt Lake City: University of Utah School of Medicine; 1989.

> Many of the skills needed by health care managers, such as leadership, making meetings productive, working through others, giving feedback, and overcoming resistance to new programs, are also important for successful development and implementation of curricula. 117 pages.

SPECIFIC REFERENCES

1. Kern DE, Grayson M, Barker LR, Roca RP, Cole KA, Roter D, Golden A. Residency training in interviewing skills and the psychosocial domain of medical practice. *J Gen Intern Med* 1989; 4:421–431.
2. American Medical Association. Section II. Essentials of accredited residencies in graduate medical education: Institutional and program requirements. In *Graduate Medical Education Directory, 1998–1999.* Chicago: American Medical Association, 1998. Pp. 25–341.
3. American College of Physicians. *Resources for Internists: 1995 Catalog.* Philadelphia: American College of Physicians; 1996. Pp. 1–28.
4. American College of Physicians Governors' Class of 1996. *Learning from Practitioners: Office-Based Teaching of Internal Medicine Residents.* Philadelphia: American College of Physicians; 1995.
5. Deutsch SL, Noble J. eds. *Community-Based Teaching: A Guide to Developing Education Programs for Medical Students and Residents in the Practitioner's Office.* Philadelphia: Pennsylvania: American College of Physicians; 1997.
6. Skeff KM, Stratos GA, Berman J, Bergen MR. Improving clinical teaching: evaluation of a national dissemination program, *Arch Intern Med* 1992; 152:1156–1161.
7. Skeff KM, Stratos GA, Bergen MR, Albright CL, Berman J, Farquhar JW, Sox HC. The Stanford faculty development program: a dissemination approach to faculty development for medical teachers; *Teaching and Learning in Medicine* 1995. 4(3): 180–187.
8. Whitman N. Overcoming resistance. In Whitman N, Weiss E, Bishop FM, eds., *Executive Skills for Medical Faculty.* Salt Lake City: University of Utah School of Medicine; 1989. Pp. 45–49.
9. Kolbe LJ, Iverson DC. Implementing comprehensive school health education: educational innovation and social change. *Health Education Quarterly* 1981; 8:63–65, 77–78.

Step 6: Evaluation and Feedback

DEFINITIONS

Evaluation, for the purposes of this book, is defined as the comparison of an object of interest to an explicit or implicit standard of acceptability (1). Feedback is defined as the provision of information about an individual's or curriculum's performance to learners, faculty, and other stakeholders in the curriculum.

IMPORTANCE

Step 6, *evaluation and feedback,* closes the loop in the curriculum development cycle. The evaluation step helps curriculum developers ask and answer the critical question, Were the goals and objectives of the curriculum met? Evaluation provides information that can be used to guide individuals and the curriculum in cycles of ongoing improvement. Evaluation results can also be used to maintain and garner support for a curriculum, to assess individual achievement, to satisfy external requirements, to document the accomplishments of curriculum developers, and to serve as a basis for presentations and publications.

It is helpful to be methodical in designing the evaluation for a curriculum to ensure that important questions are answered and relevant needs met. This chapter outlines a 10-task approach that begins with consideration of the potential users and uses of an evaluation, moves to the identification of evaluation questions and methods, proceeds to the collection of data, and ends with data analysis and reporting of results.

TASK I: IDENTIFY USERS

The first step in planning the evaluation for a curriculum is to identify the likely users of the evaluation. *Participants* in the curriculum's experience have an interest in the evaluation of their own performance and in the performance of the curriculum. Evaluation can provide feedback and motivation for continued improvement for *learners, faculty, and curriculum developers.*

Other stakeholders who have administrative responsibility for, who allocate resources to, or who are otherwise affected by the curriculum will also be interested in evaluation results. These stakeholders might include individuals in the *dean's office, hospital administrators,* the *department chair,* the *program director* for the residency program or medical student education, the *division director, other faculty* who have contributed political support or who might be in competition for limited resources, and *individuals, granting agencies, or other organizations that have contributed funds or other resources* to the curriculum. Individuals who need to make decisions about whether or not to participate in the curriculum, such as *future learners or faculty,* may also be interested in evaluation results.

To the extent that a curriculum innovatively addresses an important need or tests new educational strategies, evaluation results may also be of interest to educators from other institutions.

TASK II: IDENTIFY USES

Generic Uses

In designing an evaluation strategy for a curriculum, the curriculum developer should be aware of the generic uses of an evaluation. These generic uses can be classified along two axes, as shown in Table 7.1. The first axis refers to whether the evaluation is used to measure the performance of *individuals,* the performance of the entire *program,* or *both.* The evaluation of an individual usually involves determining whether he or she has achieved the cognitive, affective, or psychomotor objectives of a curricu-

Table 7.1.   Evaluation Types: Levels and Uses

Use	Level	
	Individual	Program
Formative	Evaluation of an individual learner or faculty member that is used to help the individual improve performance: ■ Identification of areas for improvement ■ Specific suggestions for improvement	Evaluation of a program that is used to improve program performance: ■ Identification of areas for improvement ■ Specific suggestions for improvement
Summative	Evaluation of an individual learner or faculty member that is used for judgments or decisions about the individual: ■ Verification of achievement for individual ■ Motivation of individual to maintain or improve performance ■ Certification of performance for others ■ Grades ■ Promotion	Evaluation of a program that is used for judgments or decisions about the program or program developers: ■ Judgments regarding success, efficacy ■ Decisions regarding allocation of resources ■ Motivation/recruitment of learners and faculty ■ Influencing attitudes regarding value of curriculum ■ Satisfying external requirements ■ Prestige, power, influence, promotion ■ Dissemination: presentations, publications

lum. Program evaluation usually assesses the aggregate achievements of all individuals, clinical or other outcomes, the actual processes of a curriculum, or the perceptions of learners and faculty. The second axis in Table 7.1 refers to whether an evaluation is used for *formative* purposes (to improve performance) (2), for *summative* purposes (to judge performance) (3), or for *both* purposes.

Formative individual evaluation is evaluation that provides *feedback* to an individual (usually a learner) in order to *improve* the individual's performance. This type of evaluation identifies areas for improvement and provides specific suggestions for improvement. It, therefore, also serves as an educational method (see Chapter 5).

> **EXAMPLE:** Residents during an outpatient gynecology rotation are observed doing pelvic examinations by faculty, who subsequently provide specific verbal suggestions to improve each resident's performance.

Summative individual evaluation is evaluation that measures whether specific objectives were accomplished by an individual in order to place a value on the performance of the individual. It may certify competency in a particular area, as with specialty board examinations, or may simply verify for the individual that certain objectives were achieved. In either instance, it is important to clarify criteria for the achievement of objectives or competency before the evaluation.

> EXAMPLE: At the conclusion of the gynecology rotation, each resident is observed performing a pelvic examination by a faculty preceptor with a criterion checklist, and is deemed competent or not competent in the performance of the pelvic examination.

Formative program evaluation is evaluation that provides information in order to improve a program's performance. Formative program evaluation usually takes the form of surveys of learners to obtain feedback about and suggestions for improving a curriculum. Quantitative information, such as ratings of various aspects of the curriculum, can help identify areas that need revision. Qualitative information, such as responses to open-ended questions about program strengths, program weaknesses, and suggestions for change, provides feedback in areas that may not have been anticipated and provides ideas for improvement. Information can also be obtained from faculty or other observers, such as nurses and patients. Aggregates of formative and summative individual evaluations can be used for formative program evaluation as well, in order to identify specific areas of the curriculum in need of revision.

> EXAMPLE: At the midpoint of an ambulatory clinical clerkship, students met with the clerkship director for a discussion of experiences to date. Several students discussed their discomfort about working in faculty members' offices. The clerkship director reviewed this information with faculty preceptors, who implemented measures to better integrate students into the office practices.

> EXAMPLE: After each didactic lecture of the gynecology rotation, learners were asked to complete an evaluation form, which asked them to rate the effectiveness of the speaker and the usefulness of the talk. It was discovered that residents did not learn much from the lecture on sexually transmitted diseases, because it was already covered in the Infectious Disease curriculum. The lecture was replaced.

Summative program evaluation is evaluation that measures the success of a curriculum in achieving learner objectives for all of the targeted learners, its success in achieving its process objectives, and/or its success in engaging, motivating, and pleasing its learners and faculty. In addition to quantitative data, summative program evaluation may include qualitative information about unintended barriers or unanticipated effects encountered in the program implementation. The results of summative program evaluations are often reported to others to obtain or maintain curricular time, funding, and other resources.

> EXAMPLE: At the conclusion of an ambulatory clinical clerkship, 90% of students received a passing grade in the performance of a standardized patient examination, which assessed five cognitive and nine skill objectives in the areas of history, physical examination, diagnosis, management, and counseling.

> EXAMPLE: One curricular objective of a gynecology rotation stated that internal medicine residents would subsequently integrate cervical cancer screening into their ambulatory primary care practice. One year later an audit in the residents' primary care clinic found an increase in the number of eligible women patients who had received Pap smear examinations, but most of the patients had been referred to gynecology for their examinations. Review of other evaluation results indicated that residents had achieved proficiency in performing the exami-

nations themselves. Discussion of audit results with residents revealed that the absence of a second examination room and readily available chaperones made the performance of pelvic/Pap examinations in the residents' clinic inefficient. The evaluation results were used as a stimulus for change in the operations of the medical clinic.

EXAMPLE: Summative evaluation results from a pilot curriculum in flexible sigmoidoscopy revealed a high level of learner satisfaction and provided documentation of proficiency in the procedure for all residents who had taken the curriculum. After seeing the results, the department chair created space in the ambulatory rotations of all residents for the curriculum. The division chief adjusted the schedules of the two curriculum coordinators so that they could expand the curriculum.

From the above discussion and examples, the reader may surmise that *some evaluations can be used for both summative and formative purposes.* The evaluation of specific curricular components, for example, can be used not only to judge their effectiveness but also to target areas for revision.

Specific Uses

Having identified the likely users of the evaluation and having understood the various generic uses of curriculum evaluation, the curriculum developer should consider the specific needs of different users and the specific ways in which they will put the evaluation to use (4). Specific uses for evaluation results might include the following:

- *Feedback on and improvement of individual performance:* Both learners and faculty can use the results of timely feedback (formative individual evaluation) to direct improvements in their own performances.
- *Judgments regarding individual performance:* The accomplishments of individual learners may need to be documented (summative individual evaluation) to assign grades, to demonstrate competence, or to satisfy the demands of external bodies, such as specialty boards. Assessments of individual faculty members can be used to make decisions about their continuation as curriculum faculty, as material for their promotion portfolios, and as data for teaching awards.
- *Feedback on and improvement of program performance:* Curriculum coordinators can use evaluation results (formative program evaluation) to identify parts of the curriculum that are effective and parts that are in need of improvement. Evaluation results may also provide suggestions about how parts of the curriculum could be improved.
- *Judgments regarding program success:* Summative program evaluation provides information on the degree to which a curriculum has met its various objectives and expectations.
- *Justification for the allocation of resources:* Those with administrative authority can use evaluation results (summative program evaluation) to guide and justify decisions about the allocation of resources for a curriculum and may be more likely to allocate limited resources to a curriculum if the evaluation provides evidence of success.
- *Motivation and recruitment:* Feedback on individual and program success and the identification of areas for future improvement can be motivational to faculty (formative and summative individual and program evaluation). Evidence of program success can also help in the recruitment of future faculty and learners (summative program evaluation).

- *Attitude change:* Evidence that significant change has occurred in learners (summative program evaluation) with the use of an unfamiliar method, such as videotaped reviews or role-plays, or in a previously unaccepted content area, such as psychosocial medicine, can significantly alter attitudes about the importance of such methods and content.
- *Satisfaction of external requirements:* Summative individual and program evaluation results can be used to satisfy the requirements of outside bodies, such as Residency Review Committees, and therefore will be welcomed by those who have administrative responsibility for an overall program.
- *Demonstration of popularity:* Evidence that learners (and faculty) truly enjoyed and valued their experience (summative program evaluation) may be important to educational program directors, who want to satisfy their existing trainees and recruit new ones for the program. A high degree of learner and faculty support also provides political support for a curriculum.
- *Prestige, power, promotion, and influence:* A successful program (summative program evaluation) reflects positively on its institution, department chair, division chief, overall program director, curriculum coordinator, and faculty, thereby conveying a certain degree of prestige, power, and influence. Summative program and individual evaluation data can be used as evidence of accomplishment in one's promotion portfolio.
- *Presentations, publications, and adoption of curricular components by others:* To the degree that an evaluation (summative program evaluation) provides evidence of the success (or failure) of an innovative or insufficiently studied educational program or method, the evaluation will be of interest to educators at other institutions and to publishers (see Chapter 9).

TASK III: IDENTIFY RESOURCES

The most carefully planned evaluation will fail if the resources are not available to accomplish it. Limits in resources may require prioritization of evaluation questions and changes in evaluation methods. For this reason, curriculum developers should *consider resource needs early* in the evaluation process, including *time, personnel, equipment, facilities, and funds.* Appropriate *time* should be allocated for the collection, analysis, and reporting of evaluation results. *Personnel* needs often include not only staff to help in the collection and collation of data and distribution of reports but also persons with statistical or computer expertise to help analyze the data. *Equipment and facilities* might include the appropriate computer hardware and software. *Funding* from internal or external sources is required for resources that are not otherwise available, in which case a budget and budget justification may have to be developed.

Often formal funding is not available, but informal networking will reveal potential assistance locally, for example, from computer programmers or biostatisticians interested in measurements pertinent to the curriculum, or from quality improvement personnel in a hospital interested in measuring patient outcomes. Medical schools and residency programs often have summative evaluations in place for students and residents, in the form of specialty board examinations and in-service training examinations. Specific information on learner performance in the knowledge areas addressed by these tests can be readily accessed through the department chair with little cost to the curriculum.

EXAMPLE: An objective of a two-session curriculum on talking to geriatric patients about advance directives was that residents subsequently would document discussions about advance directives with the majority of their ambulatory continuity patients who were 65 years old or older. In working through their evaluation plans, curriculum developers realized that there were insufficient resources for them to conduct follow-up audits, or even to solicit systematic follow-up self-reports. They were able, however, to have an item added to the chart audit already in existence for the residents' continuity practice experience.

TASK IV: IDENTIFY EVALUATION QUESTIONS

Most evaluation questions (5) should relate to the specific measurable learner, process, or outcome objectives of a curriculum (see Chapter 4). As described in Chapter 4, specific measurable objectives should state who will do how much (how well) of what by when. The who may refer to learners or instructors or to the program itself, if one is evaluating program activities; how much (how well) of what by when provides a standard of acceptability that is measurable. Often, in the process of writing evaluation questions and thinking through what evaluation design and methods might be able to answer a question, it becomes clear that a curricular objective needs further clarification.

EXAMPLE: An objective, as initially drafted, stated, "By the end of the curriculum, all residents will be proficient in smoking cessation counseling." In formulating the evaluation question and thinking through the evaluation methodology, it became clear to the curriculum developers that "proficient" needed to be defined operationally. In addition, they decided that they would consider the curriculum a success if 90% or more of the residents were proficient by the end of the curriculum and if there was a statistically and quantitatively significant (>25%) increase in the number of residents who were proficient by the end of the curriculum. After appropriate revisions in the objective, the evaluation questions became: "By the end of the curriculum, what percentage of residents have achieved a passing score on the curriculum's proficiency checklist for smoking cessation counseling, as assessed using standardized patients?" and "Has there been a statistically and quantitatively (>25%) significant increase in the number of proficient residents, as defined above, from the beginning to the end of the curriculum?"

The curriculum developer should also make sure that the evaluation question is *congruent* with the related curricular objective.

EXAMPLE: An objective of a gynecology curriculum for internal medicine residents might be that they obtain proficiency in the screening pelvic and Pap examination of asymptomatic women (a skill or competency objective). The evaluation question, "In what percentage of their eligible population of continuity practice patients do residents, postcurricularly, perform the screening and Pap examinations themselves?" is not congruent with the objective as worded, because the evaluation question addresses a performance and not a skill objective. A congruent evaluation question would be: "By the end of the curriculum, what percentage of the residents are proficient in performing a pelvic and Pap examination?" Curriculum developers may have to ask themselves whether they want to add a performance objective for the curriculum. If so, it would be appropriate for their curriculum to address, in addition to skill acquisition: attitudes, such as role perceptions; environmental factors, such as equipment, space, and available chaperones; and feedback on performance.

Often resources will limit the number of objectives for which accomplishment can be assessed. In this situation it is necessary to *prioritize and select key evaluation questions,* based upon the needs of the users and upon the feasibility of the related evaluation methodology. Sometimes several objectives can be grouped efficiently into a single evaluation question.

> **EXAMPLE:** A curriculum has cognitive, attitudinal, skill, and performance objectives related to the cost-effective management of back pain patients. The curriculum coordinators decide that what matters most is postcurricular performance and that effective performance requires achievement of the appropriate cognitive, attitudinal, and skill objectives. Their evaluation question and evaluation methodology, therefore, assesses postcurricular performance rather than knowledge, attitudes, or competence. It is assumed that, if the performance objectives are met, there has been sufficient accomplishment of the knowledge, attitude, and skill objectives.

Not all evaluation questions need to relate to explicit, written curricular objectives. Some curricular objectives are implicitly understood, but not written down, to prevent a curriculum document from becoming unwieldy. Most curriculum developers, for example, will want to *include evaluation questions that relate to the effectiveness of specific curricular components or faculty,* even when the related objectives are implicit rather than explicit.

> **EXAMPLE:** What was the perceived effectiveness of the curriculum's small-group discussions, simulated patients, clinical experiences, and required case presentations?

Sometimes, there are unexpected strengths and weaknesses in a curriculum. Sometimes, the curriculum on paper may differ from the curriculum as delivered (6). Therefore, it is almost always helpful to *include some questionnaire items that do not relate to specific curricular objectives and that are open-ended in nature.*

> **EXAMPLE:** What actually happens during the learning sessions? What issues are most frequently raised, and how are they addressed? What do learners perceive as the major strengths and weaknesses of the curriculum? How could the curriculum be improved?

TASK V: CHOOSE EVALUATION DESIGNS

Once the evaluation questions have been identified and prioritized, the curriculum developer should consider *which evaluation designs (7–10) are most appropriate to answer the evaluation questions and most feasible in terms of resources.*

An evaluation is said to possess *internal validity* (11) if it accurately assesses the impact of a specific intervention on specific subjects in a specific setting. An internally valid evaluation that is generalizable to other populations and other settings is said to possess *external validity* (11). Usually a curriculum's targeted learners and setting are predetermined for the curriculum developer. To the extent that the uniqueness of the subjects and setting can be minimized and their representativeness maximized, the external validity of the evaluation will be strengthened.

The choice of evaluation design, which is in the control of the curriculum developer, affects directly the internal validity and indirectly the external validity of an evaluation. In choosing an evaluation design, it is important to be aware of each design's strengths and limitations with respect to *factors that could threaten the internal validity of the evaluation.* These factors include history, maturation, testing, instrumentation, selection bias, dropout bias, and statistical regression (7, 8, 11). *History* refers to events or other interventions that affect subjects during the period of an evaluation. *Maturation* refers to changes within subjects that occur as a result of the passage of time rather than as a result of discrete external interventions. *Testing* refers to the effects of an initial test on subjects' performance on subsequent tests. *Instrumentation* refers to the effects that changes in raters or measurement methods, or that lack of precision in the measurement instrument, might have on obtained measurements. *Selection bias* occurs when subjects in an intervention or comparison group possess characteristics that affect the results of the evaluation, by affecting the measurements of interest or the response of subjects to the intervention. *Dropout bias* occurs when two groups being compared differ in the incidence of subjects dropping out of the evaluation. *Statistical regression* can occur when subjects have been selected on the basis of extreme scores on a test. Because of temporal variations in the performance of individuals, and because of characteristics of the test itself that result in imperfect test-retest reliability (see Task VI), subsequent scores on the test are likely to be less extreme, whether or not an educational intervention takes place. It may not be possible or feasible, in the choice of evaluation design, to prevent all of the above factors from affecting a given evaluation. However, the curriculum developer should be aware of the potential effects of these factors when choosing an evaluation design and when interpreting the results.

The most commonly used *evaluation designs* are posttest only, pretest-posttest, nonrandomized controlled pretest-posttest, randomized controlled posttest only, and randomized controlled pretest-posttest (7–10). *As the designs increase in methodologic rigor, they also increase in the amount of resources required to execute them.*

A *posttest only* design can be diagrammed as follows:

$$X - - - O$$

where X represents the curriculum or educational intervention, and O represents observations or measurements. This design permits assessment of what learners have achieved after the educational intervention, but the achievements could have been present prior to the intervention (selection bias), could have occurred as part of a natural maturation process during the period of the evaluation (maturation), or could have resulted from other interventions that took place during the evaluation period (history). The design is appropriate when the most important evaluation question is the certification of proficiency. The design is also well suited to assess participant perceptions of the curriculum, to solicit suggestions for improvement in the curriculum, and to solicit feedback on and ratings of student or faculty performance.

A *pretest-posttest* design can be diagrammed as follows:

$$O_1 - - - X - - - O_2$$

where O_1 represents the first observations or measurements, in this case before the educational intervention, and O_2 the second observations or measurements, in this case after the intervention. This design can demonstrate that changes in proficiency have occurred in learners during the course of the curriculum. However, the changes could have occurred because of factors other than the curriculum (e.g., history, maturation, testing, instrumentation).

The addition of a *control group* helps confirm that an observed change occurred because of the curriculum, particularly if the control group was *randomized*. A *pretest-posttest controlled evaluation design* can be diagrammed as follows:

$$E \quad O_1 \text{ - - - } X \text{ - - - } O_2$$
$$R$$
$$C \quad O_1 \text{ - - - - - - - } O_2$$

where E represents the experimental or intervention group, C represents the control or comparison group, and R (if present) indicates that subjects were randomized between the intervention and control groups. A *posttest only randomized controlled design* requires fewer resources, especially when the observations or measurements are difficult and resource intensive. It, however, cannot demonstrate changes in learners. Furthermore, the success of the randomization process in achieving comparability between the intervention and control group prior to the curriculum cannot be assessed. This design can be diagrammed as follows:

$$E \quad X \text{ - - - } \qquad O_1$$
$$R$$
$$C \qquad \text{ - - - } \qquad O_1$$

Evaluation designs are sometimes classified as pre-experimental, quasi-experimental, and true experimental (8, 12). *Pre-experimental designs* usually lack controls. *Quasi-experimental designs* usually include controls but lack random assignment. *True experimental designs* include both random assignment to experimental and control groups and concurrent observations or measurements in the experimental and control groups.

The advantages and disadvantages of each of the discussed evaluation designs are displayed in Table 7.2. Additional evaluation designs are possible (see General References at end of chapter).

Sometimes political or ethical considerations prohibit withholding a curriculum from some learners. This obstacle to a controlled evaluation can sometimes be overcome by delaying administration of the curriculum to the control group until after data collection has been completed for a randomized controlled evaluation.

EXAMPLE: *Controlled Evaluation without Denying the Curriculum to the Control Group.* The design for such an evaluation might be diagrammed as follows:

$$E \quad O_1 \text{ - - - } X \text{ - - - } O_2 \qquad\qquad (\text{ - - - } O_3)$$
$$R$$
$$C \quad O_1 \text{ - - - - - - - } O_2 \text{ - - - - } X \qquad (\text{ - - - } O_3)$$

Using this evaluation design, a randomized controlled evaluation is accomplished without denying the curriculum to any learner. Inclusion of additional observation points, as indicated in the parentheses, is more resource intensive but permits inclusion of all (not just half) of the learners in a noncontrolled pretest-posttest evaluation.

It is important to realize that formative evaluation and feedback may occur in an ongoing fashion during a curriculum and could be diagrammed as follows:

$$O_1 \text{ - - - } X \text{ - - - } O_2 \text{ - - - } X \text{ - - - } O_3 \text{ - - - } X \text{ - - - } O_4$$

In this situation, a formative evaluation strategy is also an educational strategy for the curriculum.

Table 7.2.   Advantages and Disadvantages of Commonly Used Evaluation Designs

Evaluation Design	Diagram	Advantages	Disadvantages
Posttest only (pre-experimental)	X - - - O	Simple Economical Can document proficiency Can document process (what happened) Can ascertain learner and faculty perceptions of efficacy and value Can elicit suggestions for improvement	Accomplishments may have been pre-existing Accomplishments may be the result of natural maturation Accomplishments may be due to factors other than the curriculum
Pretest-posttest (pre-experimental)	O_1 - - - X - - - O_2	Intermediate in complexity and cost Can demonstrate pre/post changes in cognitive, affective, and psychomotor attributes, performance, and perceptions	Accomplishments may be the result of natural maturation Accomplishments may be due to factors other than the curriculum Accomplishments could result from learning from the first test or evaluation rather than from the curriculum
Controlled pretest-posttest (quasi-experimental)	E O_1 - - - X - - - O_2 C O_1 - - - - - - - O_2	Controls for maturation, if control group equivalent Controls for the effects of measured factors, other than the curriculum Controls for learning from the test or evaluation	Complex Resource intensive Control group may not be equivalent to the experimental group, and changes could be due to differences in unmeasured factors Curriculum denied to some (see text)
Randomized controlled posttest only (true experimental)	E X - - - O_1 R C - - - O_1	Controls for maturation Controls for effects of measured and unmeasured factors Less resource intensive than a randomized controlled pretest-posttest design, while preserving the benefits of randomization	Complex Resource intensive Does not demonstrate changes in learners Totally dependent on the success of the randomization process in eliminating pretest differences in independent and dependent variables Curriculum denied to some (see text)

Table 7.2.   *(continued)*

Evaluation Design	Diagram	Advantages	Disadvantages
Randomized controlled pretest-posttest (true experimental)	E O_1 - - - X - - - O_2 R C O_1 - - - - - - O_2	Controls for maturation Controls for effects of measured and unmeasured factors Controls for the effects of testing	Most complex Most resource intensive Curriculum denied to some (see text) Depends on success of the randomization process in eliminating pretest differences in unmeasured independent and dependent variables

O = observation or measurement
X = curriculum or educational intervention
E = experimental or intervention group
C = control or comparison group
R = random allocation to experimental and control groups

TASK VI: CHOOSE MEASUREMENT METHODS AND CONSTRUCT INSTRUMENTS

The choice of measurement methods and construction of measurement instruments is a crucial step in the evaluation process because it determines the data that will be collected.

Choice of Measurement Methods

Measurement methods commonly used to evaluate individuals and programs include rating forms, self-assessment forms, essays, written or computer-interactive tests, oral examinations, questionnaires, individual interviews, group interviews/discussions, direct observation, and performance audits (13). The uses, strengths, and limitations of each of these measurement methods are displayed in Table 7.3.

As with the choice of evaluation design, *it is important to choose a measurement method that is congruent with the evaluation question* (14).

> **EXAMPLE:** A written test is an appropriate method for assessing knowledge acquisition. Direct observation, using agreed-upon standards, is an appropriate method for assessing skill attainment. Chart audit and unobtrusive observations are appropriate methods for assessing real-life performance.

It is also necessary to choose measurement methods that are *feasible in terms of available resources*. Curriculum developers usually have to make difficult decisions regarding how to spread limited resources among the problem identification, needs assessment, educational intervention, and evaluation.

> **EXAMPLE:** Global rating forms for use by faculty supervisors and self-assessment questionnaires for completion by learners provide indirect, inexpensive measures of skill attainment

Table 7.3.   Uses, Strengths, and Limitations of Commonly Used Evaluation Methods

Method	Uses	Strengths	Limitations
Rating forms	Cognitive, affective, or psychomotor attributes; real-life performance	Economical Can evaluate anything Open-ended questions can provide information for formative purposes	Subjective Rater biases Inter- and intra-rater reliability Raters frequently have insufficient data upon which to base ratings
Self-assessment forms	Cognitive, affective, psychomotor attributes; real-life performance	Economical Can evaluate anything Promotes self-assessment Useful for formative evaluation	Subjective Rater biases Agreement with objective measurements often low Limited acceptance as method of summative evaluation
Essays on respondent's experience	Attitudes, feelings, description of respondent experiences, perceived impact	Rich in texture Provides unanticipated as well as anticipated information Respondent centered	Subjective Rater biases Requires qualitative evaluation methods to analyze Focus varies from respondent to respondent
Written or computer-interactive tests	Knowledge; higher-level cognitive ability	Often economical Objective Widely accepted Essay-type questions can economically assess higher level cognitive ability	Reliability/validity vary with quality and purpose of test Constructing tests of higher-level cognitive ability, or computer-interaction tests, can be resource intensive
Oral examinations	Knowledge; higher level cognitive ability; indirect measure of affective attributes	Flexible; can follow up and explore understanding Learner centered Can be integrated into case discussions	Subjective Inter- and intra-rater reliability Faculty intensive

Table 7.3. *(continued)*

Method	Uses	Strengths	Limitations
Questionnaires	Attitudes; perceptions; suggestions for improvement	Economical	Subjective Constructing reliable and valid measures of attitudes requires time and skill
Individual interviews	Attitudes; perceptions; suggestions for improvement	Flexible; can follow up and clarify responses Respondent centered	Subjective Rater biases Constructing reliable and valid measures of attitudes requires time and skill Requires interviewers
Group interviews/ discussions	Attitudes; perceptions; suggestions for improvement	Flexible: can follow up and develop/ explore responses Respondent centered Efficient means of interviewing several subjects at once Group interaction can enrich or deepen information Can be integrated into teaching sessions	Subjective Requires skilled interviewer or facilitator to control group interaction and minimize facilitator influence on responses Does not yield quantitative information Information may not be representative of all participants
Direct observation	Skills; performance	Firsthand data Can provide immediate feedback to the observed Development of standards, use of observation checklists, and training of observers can increase reliability and validity	Rater biases Inter- and intra-rater reliability Personnel intensive Unless observation is covert, assesses capability rather than real life performance
Performance audits	Record keeping; provision of recorded care (e.g., tests ordered, provision of preventive care measures, prescribed treatments)	Objective Reliability and accuracy can be measured and enhanced by the use of standards and the training of raters Unobtrusive	Dependent on what is reliably recorded; much care is not Dependent on available, organized records or data sources

and real-life performance. These forms, however, are subject to numerous rating biases. Direct observation or audits that use trained raters and agreed-upon standards are more reliable and valid methods for measuring skills and performance than are global rating forms, but they also require more resources. There is little point in using the latter measurement methods, however, if their use would drain resources that are critically important for achieving a successful educational intervention.

Construction of Measurement Instruments

Most evaluations will require the construction of curriculum specific measurement instruments such as tests, rating forms, interview schedules, or questionnaires.

The *methodologic rigor* with which the instruments are constructed and administered affects the reliability, validity, and, unfortunately, cost of the evaluation. Formative evaluations generally require the least rigor; summative individual and program evaluation for internal use, an intermediate level of rigor; and summative individual and program evaluation for external use (e.g., certification of competence or publication of evaluation results), the most rigor. When a high degree of methodologic rigor is required, it is worth exploring whether there is an *already existing measurement instrument* (15–19) that is appropriate in terms of content, reliability, validity, feasibility, and cost. When a methodologically rigorous instrument must be constructed specifically for a curriculum, it is wise to seek *advice or mentorship from individuals with expertise in designing such instruments*.

A useful first step in constructing measurement instruments is to determine the desired *content*. For assessments of curricular impact, this first step involves the identification of independent variables and dependent variables. *Independent variables* are factors that could explain or predict the curriculum's outcomes (e.g., the curriculum itself, previous or concurrent training, environmental factors). *Dependent variables* are program outcomes (e.g., knowledge or skill attainment, real-life performance, clinical outcomes). To keep the measurement instruments from becoming unwieldy, it is prudent to focus on a few dependent variables that are most relevant to the main evaluation questions and, similarly, to focus on the independent variables that are most likely to be related to the curriculum's outcomes.

Next, attention must be devoted to the *format* of the instruments. In determining the acceptable *length* for a measurement instrument, methodologic concerns and the desire to be comprehensive must be balanced against constraints in the amount of curricular time allotted for evaluation, imposition on respondents, and concerns about response rate. Individual items should be worded and displayed in a manner that is *clear and unambiguous*. *Response scales* (e.g., "true"-"false"; "strongly disagree," "disagree," "neither agree nor disagree," "agree," "strongly agree") should make sense relative to the question asked. There is no consensus about whether it is preferable for response scales to have middle points or not (e.g., "neither agree nor disagree") or to have an even or odd number of response categories. In general, four to seven response categories permit greater flexibility in data analysis than two or three do. It is important for the instrument as a whole to be *user-friendly*. This is done by organizing the instrument in a manner that facilitates quick understanding and efficient recording of responses. It is desirable for the instrument to *engage* the interest of respondents.

Before using an instrument for evaluation purposes, it is almost always important to *pilot* it on a convenient audience. Audience feedback can provide important information about the instrument: how it is likely to be perceived by respondents; acceptable length;

clarity of individual items; user-friendliness of the overall format; and specific ways in which the instrument could be improved.

Reliability, Validity, and Bias

Because measurement instruments are never perfect, the data they produce is never absolutely accurate. An understanding of potential threats to accuracy is helpful to the curriculum coordinator in planning the evaluation and in reporting results and is helpful to the users of evaluation reports in interpreting results.

Reliability (20, 21) refers to the consistency or reproducibility of measurements. Ideally, measurements should be the same when repeated by the same person (*intrarater reliability*) or made by different persons (*interrater reliability*). Intra- or interrater reliability can be assessed by the percentage agreement between raters or by statistics such as kappa (22), which correct for chance agreement. Other forms of reliability include stability, equivalence, and homogeneity. *Stability,* or *test-retest reliability,* is the degree to which the same test produces the same results when repeated under the same conditions. *Equivalence,* or *alternate-form reliability* is the degree to which alternate forms of the same measurement instrument produce the same result. This form of reliability is of particular relevance in pre/post test evaluations, when test-specific learning related to test taking could occur, independent of the curricular intervention. In such circumstances, it is desirable to use equivalent but different tests or alternative forms of the same test. *Homogeneity* is the extent to which various items legitimately team together to measure a single characteristic, such as a desired attitude. Homogeneity can be assessed by using the statistic called Cronbach's (or coefficient) alpha (23), which is basically the average of the correlations of each item in a scale to the total score. A complex characteristic, however, could have several dimensions. In this situation, the technique of factor analysis (24) can be used to help separate the different dimensions. When there is a need to assess the reliability of an important measure but a lack of statistical expertise among curricular faculty, statistical consultation is advisable.

> **EXAMPLE:** *Homogeneity.* A group of educators from several institutions worked together to develop a computer-interactive case-based test to assess three cognitive areas: (a) knowledge of facts necessary for the appropriate management of two common medical disorders; (b) clinical decision making that incorporates the use of sensitivity, specificity, predictive values for diagnostic strategies, known efficacy and complications for treatment options, and patient preferences; and (c) cost-effectiveness of decisions in relation to outcomes. Factor analysis was able to identify separate generic clinical decision making and cost-effectiveness dimensions. However, there was not a single knowledge dimension. Knowledge split into two separate factors, each of which was specific to one of the two medical disorders. So did disease-specific clinical decision making, which required knowledge that was not provided in the test. Cronbach's alpha was used to assess homogeneity among items that contributed to each of the six dimensions or factors. There was a large number of items for each dimension. Those items that had low correlation with the overall score for each dimension were considered for elimination.

Validity (20, 21) refers to whether a measurement instrument truly measures what it is supposed to measure. There are several approaches to evaluating an instrument's validity. *Face, surface, or content validity* is the degree to which an instrument seems accurately to represent the skill or characteristic it is designed to measure, based upon people's experience and available knowledge. This form of validity can be enhanced by conducting an appropriate literature review to identify the most relevant content and by revising the instrument until a reasonable degree of consensus about its face validity is achieved among knowledgeable reviewers.

> **EXAMPLE:** *Face Validity.* A test that is intended to measure the knowledge of students who are completing a rotation in general surgery could be reviewed by a group of faculty and practicing surgeons to ensure that the test items cover content relevant to the practice of general surgery. It could also be reviewed by some emergency medicine and primary care physicians to ensure that the test items cover surgical principles relevant to the practice of general medicine.

Criterion-related validity includes concurrent validity and predictive validity. *Concurrent validity* is the degree to which a measurement instrument produces the same results as another accepted or proven instrument that measures the same parameters. *Predictive validity* is the degree to which a measure accurately predicts expected outcomes (e.g., a measure of attitudes toward preventive care should correlate significantly with preventive care behaviors).

> **EXAMPLE:** *Concurrent Validity.* The clinical skills of residents can be assessed by using self-ratings, faculty ratings, or an examination that includes a standardized patient. The faculty members agree that the standardized patient examination has the greatest face validity, but they would like if possible to substitute one of the less costly methods. On literature review, however, the first two measures were found to correlate poorly with scores on a standardized patient examination (25).

> **EXAMPLE:** *Predictive Validity.* Many residency programs use in-training examinations to assess the knowledge base of their residents. The results of the in-training examinations should be predictive of how well individuals will perform on their certifying examinations. Program directors rely on the predictive validity of the in-training examinations when they counsel residents with low scores on specific subsections.

Construct validity refers to whether a measurement instrument performs as would theoretically be expected in groups that are known to possess or not possess the attribute being measured, or in comparison to tests that are known to measure the same attribute (high correlation) or different attributes (low correlation).

> **EXAMPLE:** *Construct Validity.* An instrument that measures clinical reasoning ability would be expected to distinguish between individuals rated by faculty as high and low in clinical reasoning and judgment. Scores on the instrument would be expected to correlate significantly with grades on an evidence-based case presentation, but not with measures of compassion.

Internal and external validity is discussed above in reference to evaluation designs (Task V). It is worth noting here that the reliability and validity of an evaluation's measurement instruments affect the internal validity of the overall evaluation.

Planners and users of curriculum evaluations should be aware of various rating biases, particularly when global rating forms are being used by untrained raters to assess learner or faculty performance (26). Rating biases can affect both an instrument's reliability and validity. *Errors of leniency or harshness* occur when raters consistently rate higher than is accurate (e.g., Garrison Keillor's *Lake Wobegone,* where "all the women are strong, all the men are good looking, and all the children are above average") or lower than is accurate (e.g., judging junior generalist physicians against standards appropriate to senior specialist physicians). The *error of central tendency* refers to the tendency of raters to avoid extremes. The *halo effect* occurs when individuals who perform well in one area or relate particularly well to others are rated inappropriately high in other, often unobserved, areas of performance. *Attribution error* occurs when raters make inferences about why individuals behave as they do and then, based on these inferences, rate these individuals in areas that are unobserved.

> **EXAMPLE:** *Attribution Error.* A student who consistently arrives late and does not contribute actively to group discussions is assumed to be lazy and unreliable. She is rated low on motivation. The individual has a problem with child care and is quiet. But she has done all the required reading, has been active in defining her own learning needs, and has independently pursued learning resources beyond those provided in the course syllabus.

When necessary, *rater biases can be reduced and interrater and intrarater reliability can be improved by training* those who are performing the ratings.

The above discussion of reliability and validity pertains to quantitative measurements. Frequently *qualitative information* is also gathered to enrich and help explain the quantitative data that has been obtained. *Qualitative evaluation methods* are also used to explore in depth the processes and impact of a curriculum and to develop hypotheses about the way in which a curriculum works and about the effects of a curriculum.

> **EXAMPLE:** Questionnaires may ask for comments next to quantitative ratings. Respondents may be asked to list strengths, weaknesses, and suggestions for improving an entire curriculum or its components. Essays or open-ended interviews may be used to assess how a curriculum has affected participants.

When qualitative measurements are used as the primary methods of evaluating a curriculum, there may be concern about their accuracy and about the interpretation of conclusions that are drawn from the data. While a discussion of the accuracy of qualitative measurement methods is beyond the scope of this book, it is worth noting that there are concepts in qualitative research that parallel the quantitative research concepts of reliability and validity. *Trustworthiness, credibility, transferability, dependability,* and *confirmability* are concepts that can be used to assess the reproducibility and truthfulness of qualitative evaluation findings (27–29).

Because all measurement instruments are subject to threats to their reliability and validity, the ideal evaluation strategy will employ *multiple measurements that include several different measurement methods and several different raters.* When all results are similar, the findings are said to be *robust,* and one can be reasonably comfortable about their validity.

TASK VII: ADDRESS ETHICAL CONCERNS

More than any other step in the curriculum development process, evaluation is likely to raise ethical concerns. These concerns usually fall into the following categories: confidentiality, access, consent, resource allocation, and potential impact of the evaluation. It is wise for curriculum developers to anticipate ethical concerns and address them in planning the evaluation. In addressing important ethical concerns, it can be helpful to obtain input both from the involved parties, such as learners and faculty, and from those with administrative oversight for the overall program. Institutional policies and procedures, external guidelines, and consultation with uninvolved parties can also provide assistance.

Confidentiality, Access, and Consent

Concerns about confidentiality, access, and consent usually relate to those who are being evaluated. Decisions about confidentiality must be made regarding who should have access to an individual's evaluations, especially in areas of particular sensitivity such as attitudes, interpersonal skills, and teaching ability. Concerns are magnified when feasibility considerations have resulted in the use of measurement methods of limited reliability and validity and when there is a need for those reviewing the evaluations to understand these limitations.

The decision also has to be made about whether any evaluators should be granted confidentiality (evaluator is unknown to the evaluated but can be identified by someone else) or anonymity (evaluator is known to no one). This concern usually pertains to individuals in subordinate positions (e.g., students, employees) who have been asked to evaluate those in authority over them and who might be subject to retaliation for an unflattering evaluation. Anonymous raters may be more open and honest but may also be less responsible in criticizing the person being rated.

Finally, it is necessary to decide whether those being evaluated need to provide informed consent for the evaluation process. Even if a separate formal consent for the evaluation is not required, decisions need to be made regarding the extent to which those being evaluated will be informed about the evaluation methods being used; about the strengths and limitations of the evaluation methods; about the potential users of the evaluation (e.g., deans, program directors, board review committees); about the uses to which evaluation results will be put (e.g., formative purposes, grades, certification of proficiency for external bodies); about the location of evaluation results, their confidentiality, and methods for ensuring confidentiality; and, finally, about the evaluation results themselves. Which evaluation results will be shared with whom, and how will that sharing take place? Will collated or individual results be shared? Will individual results be shared by mailings or through facilitated feedback to individuals?

Resource Allocation

The use of resources for one purpose may mean that fewer resources are available for other purposes. The curriculum developer may need to ask whether the allocation of resources for a curriculum is fair and whether the allocation is likely to result in the most overall good. A strong evaluation could drain resources from other curriculum development steps. It is, therefore, appropriate to think about the effect of resource allocation on learners, faculty, curriculum coordinators, and other stakeholders in the curriculum.

> **EXAMPLE:** A controlled evaluation may deny an educational intervention to some learners. This consequence may be justified if the efficacy of the intervention is widely perceived as questionable and if there is consensus about the need to resolve the question through a controlled evaluation.
>
> On the other hand, allocation of resources to an evaluation effort that is important for a faculty member's academic advancement, but that diverts needed resources from learners or other faculty, is ethically problematic.
>
> There may also be concerns about the allocation of resources for the different evaluation purposes. How much should be allocated for formative purposes to help learners and the curriculum improve, and how much should be allocated for summative purposes to ensure competence for the public or to develop evidence of programmatic success for the curriculum developers or institution?

Potential Impact

The evaluation may have an impact on learners, faculty, curriculum developers, other stakeholders, and the curriculum itself. It is helpful to think about how an evaluation might be used and about whether the evaluation is likely to result in more good than harm. An evaluation that lacks methodologic rigor because of resource limitations could lead to false conclusions, improper interpretation, and harmful use. It is, therefore, important to ensure that (a) the uses to which an evaluation is put are appropriate for its degree of methodologic rigor, (b) the necessary degree of methodologic rigor is maintained over time, and (c) the users are informed about an evaluation's methodologic limitations as well as its strengths.

EXAMPLE: *Individual Evaluations That Are Insufficiently Accurate for Summative Evaluation.* A residency director is interested in using evaluations from a curriculum for certification of learner competence. Because the curriculum coordinator does not have the resources to develop individual summative evaluations of sufficient accuracy, the coordinator decides to use the observational evaluations that are feasible for formative purposes. The evaluations are discussed in an interactive way with learners during educational sessions to help learners improve their skills. However, because the evaluations lack sufficient interrater reliability and accuracy, the evaluation results are neither kept, nor used for summative evaluation purposes, nor entered into the residents' records where others would have access to them.

EXAMPLE: *Inability to Conduct a Sufficiently Accurate Summative Program Evaluation.* Curriculum developers who are introducing a needed curriculum to an institution, where there is much competition for resources, would like to confirm the curriculum's efficacy, which has been demonstrated elsewhere. Because the small numbers of learners available for the first curricular cycle is small and resources are too limited to ensure the reliability of measurements, the developers decide that they cannot conduct an evaluation of sufficient power and methodologic rigor to demonstrate a positive impact even if it occurred. They feel that more harm than good could come from such an attempt. They, therefore, decide to focus their evaluation on formative learner and program evaluation and on an assessment of learner satisfaction with the program. This approach is likely to help them improve the curriculum and secure the time and resources necessary for curricular expansion. An objective evaluation of sufficient power and rigor to assess program efficacy might then be feasible.

EXAMPLE: *Informing Users about Methodologic Limitations of an Evaluation Method.* Global rating forms that are placed in individuals' records are accompanied by a listing of the limitations of these forms, information on the wide variety of interrater reliability in the institution, and advice on how to interpret the forms.

TASK VIII: COLLECT DATA

Sufficient data must be collected to ensure a useful analysis. Low response rates or failure to collect important evaluation data can seriously compromise the value of an evaluation. Excessive data collection or inefficiencies in data collection can consume valuable resources.

Response Rates and Efficiency

While the evaluation design dictates when data should be collected relative to an intervention, curriculum coordinators usually have flexibility with respect to the precise time, place, and manner of data collection. Data collection can therefore be planned to maximize response rates and efficiency.

Response rates can be boosted and the need for follow-up reduced when data collection is built into scheduled learner activities. Response rates can also be increased if completion of an evaluation by a learner is necessary to achieve needed credit.

> **EXAMPLE:** During a curriculum's last educational session, fifteen minutes were set aside for learners to complete a questionnaire evaluating the curriculum. Follow-up was necessary for only two learners who missed the final session but who needed to complete the questionnaire to obtain credit for the course.

Sometimes an evaluation method can be designed to serve also as an educational method. This strategy reduces imposition on the learner and uses curriculum personnel efficiently.

> **EXAMPLE:** Interactions between faculty participants and a standardized learner were videotaped at the beginning and end of a five-session faculty development workshop. For educational purposes, the videotapes were reviewed with participants during the sessions. Later they were reviewed in a blinded fashion by trained raters as part of a pre-post evaluation.

Occasionally, data collection can be incorporated into already scheduled evaluation activities.

> **EXAMPLE:** A multiple-station examination was used to assess student accomplishments at the end of a clinical clerkship in emergency medicine. Curriculum developers for a minicurriculum on universal precautions and follow-up of needle sticks were granted a station for a computer interactive evaluation during the examination.

> **EXAMPLE:** Developers of a geriatric curriculum on advance directives convinced the director of the residents' ambulatory continuity clinic experience to include documentation of discussions about advance directives as an item in the residents' yearly chart audit.

Impact on Instrument Design

What data is collected is determined by the choice of measurement instruments (see Task VI). However, the design of measurement instruments needs to be tempered by the process of data collection. Response rates for mailed questionnaires will fall as their length and complexity increase. The amount of time and resources that have been allocated for data collection cannot be exceeded without affecting learners, faculty, or other priorities.

> **EXAMPLE:** If 15 minutes of curricular time are allocated for evaluation, a measurement instrument that requires 30 minutes to complete will intrude upon other activities and is likely to reduce participant cooperation.

Assignment of Responsibility

Measurement instruments must be distributed, collected, and stored. Nonrespondents require follow-up. While different individuals may distribute or administer measurement instruments within scheduled sessions, it is usually wise to delegate overall responsibility for data collection to one person.

> **EXAMPLE:** A faculty member with a particular interest in evaluation was named evaluation coordinator for a curriculum. He worked with the curriculum secretary to ensure that measure-

ment instruments were distributed, collected, and stored in a reliable manner. Nonrespondents were consistently pursued by the curriculum secretary.

TASK IX: ANALYZE DATA

After the data has been collected, it needs to be analyzed. *Data analysis, however, should be planned at the same time that evaluation questions are being identified and measurement instruments developed.*

Relation to Evaluation Questions

The nature of evaluation questions will determine the type of statistical approach required to answer them. Questions related to participant perceptions of a curriculum, or related to the percentage of learners who achieved a specific objective, generally require only descriptive statistics. Questions about changes in learners generally require more sophisticated tests of statistical significance.

Statistical considerations may also influence the choice of evaluation questions. A *power analysis* (30) is a statistical method for estimating the ability of an evaluation to detect a statistically significant relation between an outcome measure (dependent variable) and a potential determinant of the outcome (independent variable, such as exposure to a curriculum). The power analysis can be used to determine whether a curriculum has a sufficient number of learners to justify an assessment of the statistical significance of its effects. Sometimes there are limitations in the evaluator's statistical expertise and in the resources available for statistical consultation. Evaluation questions can then be worded in a way that at least ensures *congruence* between the questions and the analytic methods that will be employed.

> **EXAMPLE:** To avoid having to apply tests of statistical significance, an evaluation question was changed from "Does the curriculum result in a statistically significant improvement in the proficiency of its learners in skill X?" to "What percentage of learners improve or achieve proficiency in skill X by the end of the curriculum?"

When the curriculum evaluation involves a very large number of learners, analysis could reveal a statistically significant but an educationally meaningless effect on learners. The latter consideration might prompt curriculum evaluators to develop an evaluation question that addresses the magnitude as well as the statistical significance of any impact.

Relation to Measurement Instruments

The measurement instrument determines the type of data that is collected. *The type of data, in turn, helps determine the type of statistical test that is appropriate to analyze the data* (31) (see below). *Categorical data* is data that fits into discrete categories. It can be divided into nominal and ordinal data. *Nominal data* fits into discrete nonordered categories (e.g., sex, race, eye color, exposure or not to an intervention). *Ordinal data* fits into discrete but inherently ordered or hierarchical categories (e.g., grades A, B, C, D, F; highest educational level completed: grade school, high school, college, post-college degree program; response categories such as "strongly disagree," "disagree," "agree," "strongly agree"). *Numerical data* has meaning on a numerical scale. Numerical data can be continuous (e.g., age, weight, height) or discrete (e.g., number of procedures performed, number of sessions attended).

Data analysis considerations may affect the design of the measurement instrument. When a computer is being used, the first step in data analysis is *data entry.* In this situation, it is helpful to construct one's measurement instruments in a way that facilitates data entry, such as the precoding of responses. If one prefers to use a specific test for statistical significance, one needs to ensure that the appropriate type of data is collected.

Choice of Statistical Methods

As indicated above, the choice of statistical method depends upon the evaluation question as well as the type of data collected. *Descriptive statistics* are sufficient to answer questions about participant perceptions, distribution of characteristics and responses, and percentage of change or achievement. For all types of data, a display of the percentages or proportions in each response category is helpful. Medians and ranges are sometimes useful in characterizing ordinal as well as numerical data. Means and standard deviations are reserved for describing numerical data. Ordinal data can sometimes be converted to numerical data so that means and standard deviations can be applied.

> **EXAMPLE:** Curriculum evaluators found it useful to convert the following response categories to numerical data so that responses could be summarized by means: "not at all," 0; "a little," 1; "a moderate amount," 2; "a lot," 3; "completely," 4.

Statistical tests of significance are required to answer questions about the statistical significance of changes in individual learners or groups of learners and of associations between various characteristics. *Parametric statistics,* such as t-tests, analysis of variance, regression, and Pearson correlation analysis, are appropriate for numerical data. Parametric tests assume that the data are "normally" distributed in a bell-shaped curve around the mean but are robust enough to tolerate some deviation from this assumption. Sometimes ordinal data can be converted to numerical data (see example above) to permit the use of parametric statistics. *Nonparametric statistics,* such as chi-square, Wilcoxon rank-sum test, Spearman's correlation statistic, and nonparametric versions of analysis of variance, are appropriate for small sample sizes, categorical, and non-normally distributed data. Computer programs are available that can perform parametric and nonparametric tests on the same data. This approach can provide a check, when numerical data do not satisfy all of the assumptions for parametric tests.

Curriculum developers have varying degrees of statistical expertise. Those developers with modest levels of expertise and limited resources (the majority) may choose to keep data analysis simple. They can consult textbooks (32, 33) on how to perform simple statistical tests, such as t-tests, chi-squares, and the Wilcoxon rank sum test. These tests, especially for small sample sizes, can be performed by hand or with a calculator and do not require access to computer programs. Sometimes, however, the needs of users will require more sophisticated approaches. Often there are individuals within or beyond one's institution who can provide statistical consultation at limited or no expense. The curriculum developer will use the statistician's time most efficiently when the evaluation questions are clearly stated and the key independent and dependent variables are clearly defined.

TASK X: REPORT RESULTS

The final step in evaluation is the reporting and distributing of results (34). In planning evaluation reports, it is helpful to think of the *needs of users.*

The *timeliness* of reports can be crucial. Individual learners benefit from the immediate feedback of formative evaluation results, so that the information can be processed while the learning experience is still fresh and can be used to enhance subsequent learning within the curriculum. Evaluation results are helpful to faculty and curriculum planners when the results are received in time to prepare for the next curricular cycle. Important decisions, such as the allocation of educational resources for the coming year, may be influenced by the timely, but not late, reporting of evaluation results. External bodies, such as funding agencies or specialty boards, may impose deadlines for the receipt of reports.

The *format* of a report should match the needs of its users. Individual learners, faculty members, and curriculum developers may want detailed evaluation reports pertaining to their particular (or the curriculum's) performance—reports that include all relevant quantitative and qualitative data provided by the measurement instruments. Administrators, deans, and department chairs may prefer brief reports that provide background information on the curriculum and that synthesize the evaluation information relevant to their respective needs. External bodies and publishers (see Chapter 9: Dissemination) may specify the format they expect for a report.

It is always desirable to *display results in a succinct and clear manner.* Collated results can be enhanced by the addition of descriptive statistics, such as percentage distributions, means, medians, and standard deviations. Other results can be displayed in a clear and efficient manner in tables, graphs, or figures. Specific examples can help explain and bring to life summaries of qualitative data.

CONCLUSION

Evaluation is not the final step in curriculum planning but is one that affects and should evolve in concert with other steps in the curriculum development process (see also Chapter 1). It provides important information that helps a program and individuals to improve their performances. It provides information that facilitates judgments and decisions about individuals and a curriculum. A stepwise approach can help ensure an evaluation that meets the needs of its users and that balances methodologic rigor with feasibility.

QUESTIONS

For the curriculum you are coordinating, planning, or would like to be planning, please answer the following:

1. Who will be the *users* of your curriculum?

2. What are their needs? *How will evaluation results be used?*

3. What *resources* are available for evaluation, in terms of *time, personnel, equipment, facilities, funds, and existing data?*

4. Identify one to three critical *evaluation questions.* Are they *congruent* with the objectives of your curriculum? Do either the objectives or evaluation questions need to be changed?

5. Name and diagram the most appropriate *evaluation design* for each evaluation question, considering both methodologic rigor and feasibility (see Table 7.2 and text).

6. Choose the most appropriate *measurement methods* for the evaluation you are designing above (see Table 7.3). Are the measurement methods *congruent* with the evaluation questions (i.e., Are you measuring the correct items)? Would it be *feasible* for you, given available resources, to construct and administer the required measurement instruments? If not, do you need to revise the evaluation questions or choose other evaluation methods?

7. What *ethical issues* are likely to be raised by your evaluation in terms of confidentiality, access, consent, resource allocation, potential impact or other concerns?

8. Consider the *data collection* process. *Who will be responsible* for data collection? How can the data be collected so that *resource use* is minimized and *response rate* is maximized? Are data collection considerations likely to influence the *design of your measurement instruments?*

9. How will the data that is collected be *analyzed*? Given your evaluation questions, are *descriptive statistics* sufficient or are *tests of statistical significance* required? Is a *power analysis* desirable? Will statistical consultation be required?

10. List the goals, content, format, and time frame of the various *evaluation reports* you envision, given the needs of the users (refer to Questions 1 and 2). How will you ensure that the reports are completed?

CONGRATULATIONS! You have read and thought about six steps critical to curriculum development. At this point it may be worthwhile rereading Chapter 1: Overview to review briefly the six steps and to reflect upon how they interact.

REMINDER: In the spirit of evaluation and feedback, we would appreciate your completing and returning the form at the end of the book.

GENERAL REFERENCES

Comprehensive

Fink A. *Evaluation Fundamentals: Guiding Health Programs, Research, and Policy.* Newbury Park, Calif.: Sage Publications; 1993.
   This is a reader-friendly, basic, comprehensive reference on program evaluation with examples from the health and social science fields. 199 pages.

Green LW, Lewis FM. *Measurement and Evaluation in Health Education and Health Promotion.* Palo Alto, Calif.: Mayfield Publishing; 1986.
   This is a clearly written, comprehensive text, with examples from community health and patient educa-

tion programs and with easy applicability to medical education programs. Both quantitative and qualitative methods are included. 411 pages.

Herman JL, ed. *Program Evaluation Kit.* 2d ed. Newbury Park, Calif.: Sage Publications; 1987.
This package comprises a user-friendly series of nine handbooks written by various authors, particularly useful for medical educators who are new to the field of evaluation. The first book is an evaluator's handbook that covers evaluation framework and kinds of evaluation; the other eight are how to manuals: how to focus an evaluation, how to design an evaluation, how to use qualitative methods in evaluation, how to assess program implementation, how to measure attitudes, how to measure performance and use tests, how to analyze data, and how to communicate findings. The nine books range from 92 to 176 pages in length.

Whitman NA, Cockayne TW. *Evaluating Medical School Courses: A User-Centered Handbook.* Salt Lake City: University of Utah, School of Medicine; 1984.
This brief handbook was written to help in planning and implementing the evaluation of medical school courses, with an emphasis on making the evaluation pertinent to the various evaluation users. The book also introduces the concept of metaevaluation (evaluating your evaluations). 35 pages.

Windsor R, Baranowski T, Clark N, Cutter G. *Evaluation of Health Promotion and Education Programs.* Palo Alto, Calif.: Mayfield Publishing; 1984.
This book was written for health professionals who are responsible for planning, implementing, and evaluating health education or health promotion programs, and has direct applicability to medical education. Especially useful are the chapters on process evaluation, program effectiveness evaluation, program data analysis, and cost-effectiveness analysis. 366 pages.

Measurement

Case SM, Swanson DB. *Constructing Written Test Questions for the Basic and Clinical Sciences.* Philadelphia: National Board of Medical Examiners; 1996.
This book was written for medical school educators who need to construct and interpret flawlessly written test questions. There are frequent examples. 115 pages.

Fink A, ed. *The Survey Kit.* 9 vols. Thousand Oaks, Calif.: Sage Publications, 1995.
This package comprises nine user-friendly, practical handbooks about various aspects of surveys both for the novice and for those who are more experienced and who want a refresher reference. The first book is an overview of the survey method. The other handbooks are "how to" manuals on asking survey questions; conducting self-administered and mail surveys; conducting interviews by telephone, in person, and by mail; designing surveys; sampling for surveys; measuring reliability and validity; analyzing survey data; and reporting on surveys. The nine books range from 73 to 223 pages in length.

Gronlund NE. *How to Make Achievement Tests and Assessments.* 5th ed. Boston: Allyn and Bacon; 1993.
This book was written for teachers without previous knowledge of measurement or statistics. The emphasis of this book is on test planning, item writing (including multiple choice, true-false, short answer, and essay questions), test assembly, test administration, and interpretation of test results. Ways to build in reliability and validity during test construction are included. 181 pages.

Miller DC. *Handbook of Research Design and Social Measurement.* Newbury Park, Calif.: Sage Publications; 1991.
The most useful part of this textbook is the 250 pages of Part 6, selected sociometric scales and indexes to measure social variables. Scales in the following areas are discussed: social status; group structure and dynamics; social indicators; measures of organizational structure; morale and job satisfaction; scales of attitudes, values, and norms; personality measurements; and many others. 704 pages.

Norman G, Shannon S, eds. *Evaluation Methods: A Resource Handbook.* Hamilton, Ontario: The Program for Educational Development, McMasters University; 1995.
This is a practical, well-written handbook on evaluation methods for assessing the performance of medical students. Reliability and validity issues are discussed for each evaluation method, including summary

reports and ratings; oral examinations; written tests; performance tests; self- and peer assessments; assessment of problem-solving, psychomotor, communication, critical appraisal skills; and evaluation of bioethics and professional behavior. 119 pages.

Evaluation Designs

Campbell DT, Stanley JC. *Experimental and Quasi-Experimental Designs for Research.* Chicago: Rand McNally; 1963.

This is a succinct, classic text on research/evaluation designs for educational programs. 84 pages.

Cook TD, Campbell DT. *Quasi Experimentation: Design and Analysis Issues for Field Settings.* Chicago: Rand McNally; 1979.

This is also a classic, but in-depth, text and is a follow-up to Campbell and Stanley's book. The book contains thorough discussions of causal inference and types of validity. 405 pages.

Qualitative Evaluation

Crabtree B, Miller W, eds. *Doing Qualitative Research.* Vol. 3 of *Research Methods for Primary Care.* Newbury Park, Calif.: Sage Publications; 1992.

This readable book focuses on qualitative research in primary care, with many examples. Chapter 1 puts qualitative studies into a taxonomy of research approaches and defines terms. Data collection and analysis strategies are discussed, including audio- and videotape analysis. 276 pages.

Denzin NK, Lincoln YS. *Handbook of Qualitative Research.* Thousand Oaks, Calif.: Sage Publications; 1994.

This is a comprehensive text, useful as a reference to look up particular topics. 643 pages.

Patton M. *Qualitative Evaluation and Research Methods.* 2d ed. Newbury Park, Calif.: Sage Publications; 1990.

This readable, example-filled text emphasizes strategies for generating useful and credible qualitative information for decision making. The three sections of the book cover conceptual issues in the use of qualitative methods; qualitative designs and data collection; and analysis, interpretation, and reporting of such studies. 532 pages.

Statistics

Kanji G. *100 Statistical Tests.* Newbury Park, Calif.: Sage Publications; 1993.

This work is a handy reference for the applied statistician and everyday user of statistics. An elementary knowledge of statistics is sufficient to allow the reader to follow the formulae given and carry out the tests. All 100 tests are cross-referenced to several headings. Examples are also included. 216 pages.

Norman G, Streiner D. *Biostatistics: The Bare Essentials.* St. Louis: Mosby; 1994.

This book conveys the traditional content for a statistics book in an irreverent and humorous tone, packaged for the "do-it-yourselfer." The main sections of the book include the nature of data and statistics; analysis of variance; regression and correlation; and nonparametric statistics. Three features of the book are very helpful: the computer notes at the end of each chapter that help the reader with the three most common statistical programs; highlighted important points in the text; and sample size calculations with each chapter. 260 pages.

Norman G, Streiner D. *PDQ Statistics.* Philadelphia: B.C. Decker; 1986.

This short, well-written book covers types of variables, descriptive statistics, parametric and nonparametric statistics, multivariate methods, and research designs. The authors assume that the reader has had some introductory exposure to statistics. The intent of the book is to help the reader understand the various approaches to analysis when reading/critiquing the results section of research articles. This book is very useful also for planning an analysis in order to avoid misuse and mis-interpretation of statistical tests. 172 pages.

Shott S. *Statistics for Health Professionals.* Philadelphia: W.B. Saunders Co.; 1990.
> The author states that after studying this text and working the problems, the reader should be able to select appropriate statistics for most data sets; interpret results; evaluate analyses reported in the literature; and interpret SPSS and SAS output for the common statistical procedures. 418 pages.

Siegel S, Castellan N. *Nonparametric Statistics for the Behavioral Sciences.* 2d ed. New York: McGraw-Hill; 1988.
> This is a usable text for understanding concepts or for reference. The information is organized by the characteristics of the data samples (single sample, paired samples, independent samples, measures of association, etc.). It includes examples that illustrate the application of tests to research problems. 399 pages.

SPECIFIC REFERENCES

1. Green LW, Lewis FM. *Measurement and Evaluation in Health Education and Health Promotion.* Palo Alto, Calif.: Mayfield Publishing; 1986. Pp. 171–176.
2. Green LW, Lewis FM. Formative evaluation and measures of quality. Chap. 2 in *Measurement and Evaluation in Health Education and Health Promotion.* Palo Alto, Calif.: Mayfield Publishing; 1986. Pp. 27–53.
3. Green LW, Lewis FM. *Measurement and Evaluation in Health Education and Health Promotion.* Palo Alto, Calif.: Mayfield Publishing; 1986. Pp. 120–121, 366.
4. Norman G, Shannon S, eds. *Evaluation Methods: A Resource Handbook.* The Program for Educational Development, Hamilton, Ontario: McMasters University; 1995. Pp. 4–8.
5. Fink A. Evaluation questions and standards. Chapter 2 in *Evaluation Fundamentals: Guiding Health Programs, Research, and Policy.* Newbury Park, Calif.: Sage Publications; 1993. Pp. 18–41.
6. Coles CR, Grant JG. Curriculum evaluation in medical health care education. *Medical Education* 1985; 19(5);405–422.
7. Green LW, Lewis FM. Selecting and implementing designs for evaluation. Chapter 9 in *Measurement and Evaluation in Health Education and Health Promotion.* Palo Alto, Calif.: Mayfield Publishing; 1986. Pp. 196–222.
8. Campbell DT, Stanley JC. *Experimental and Quasi-Experimental Designs for Research.* Chicago: Rand McNally; 1963.
9. Fink A. Designing program evaluations. Chapter 3 in *Evaluation Fundamentals: Guiding Health Programs, Research, and Policy.* Newbury Park, Calif.: Sage Publications; 1993. Pp. 43–66.
10. Fitz-Gibbon CT, Morris LL. *How to Design a Program Evaluation* (book number 3). In *Program Evaluation Kit.* Newbury Park, Calif.: Sage Publications; 1987. Pp. 25–127.
11. Cook TD, Campbell DT. *Quasi Experimentation: Design and Analysis Issues for Field Settings.* Boston: Houghton Mifflin; 1979. Pp. 50–79.
12. Cook TD, Campbell DT. *Quasi Experimentation: Design and Analysis Issues for Field Settings.* Chicago: Rand McNally; 1979. Pp. 95–146, 341–371.
13. Norman G, Shannon S, eds. *Evaluation Methods: A Resource Handbook.* The Program for Educational Development, Hamilton, Ontario: McMasters University; 1995. Pp. 25–118.
14. Morris LL, Fitz-Gibbon CT, Lindheim E. Determining how well a test fits the program. In *How to Measure Performance and Use Tests* (book number 7). In *Program Evaluation Kit.* Pp. 45–67.
15. Lorig K, Stewart A, Ritter P. Gonzalez V, Laurent D, Lynch, J. *Outcome Measures for Health Education and Other Health Care Interventions.* Thousand Oaks, Calif.: Sage Publications; 1996. Pp. 34–89.
16. McDowell I, Newill C. *Measuring Health: A Guide to Rating Scales and Questionnaires.* New York: Oxford University Press; 1987. Pp. 36–326.

17. Miller DC. *Handbook of Research Design and Social Measurement.* Newbury Park, Calif.: Sage Publications, 1991. Pp. 323–582.
18. Waltz CF, Strickland OL. *Measurement of Nursing Outcomes.* Vol. 1, *Measuring Client Outcomes;* Vol. 3, *Measuring Clinical Skills and Professional Development in Education and Practice.* New York: Springer Publishing; 1990. Vol. 1, pp. 3–537; Vol. 3, pp. 30–348.
19. Henerson ME, Morris LL, Fitz-Gibbon CT. Finding an existing measure. In *How to Measure Attitudes* (book number 6). In Herman JL, ed., *Program Evaluation Kit.* 2d ed. Newbury Park, Calif.: Sage Publications; 1987. Pp. 39–56, 178–181.
20. Windsor R, Baranowski T, Clark N, Cutter G. *Evaluation of Health Promotion and Education Programs.* Palo Alto, Calif.: Mayfield Publishing; 1984. Pp. 182–185, 185–188, 189–195.
21. Fink A. *Evaluation Fundamentals: Guiding Health Programs, Research, and Policy.* Newbury Park, Calif.: Sage Publications, 1993. Pp. 110–114.
22. Siegel S, Castellan N. *Nonparametric Statistics,* 2d ed. New York: McGraw-Hill; 1988. Pp. 284–291, 310–311.
23. Hatcher L, Stepanski EJ. *A Step-by-Step Approach to Using the SAS System for Univariate and Multivariate Statistics.* Cary, N.C.: SAS Institute; 1994. Pp. 505–516.
24. Norman G, Streiner D. *Biostatistics: The Bare Essentials.* St. Louis: Mosby; 1994. Pp. 129–142.
25. Stillman P, Swanson D, Regan MB et al. Assessment of clinical skills of residents utilizing standardized patients: A follow-up study and recommendations for application. *Ann Intern Med* 1991; 114:393–401.
26. Neufeld VR, Norman GR. *Assessing Clinical Competence.* New York: Springer Publishing; 1985. Pp. 28–138.
27. Crabtree B, Miller W. *Doing Qualitative Research.* Vol. 3 of *Research Methods for Primary Care.* Newbury Park, Calif.: Sage Publications; 1992. Pp. 232–235.
28. Marshall C, Rossman G. *Designing Qualitative Research.* Newbury Park, Calif.: Sage Publications; 1989. Pp. 144, 153.
29. Denzin NK, Lincoln YS, eds. *Handbook of Qualitative Research.* Thousand Oaks, Calif.: Sage Publications; 1994. P. 114.
30. Shott S. *Statistics for Health Professionals.* Philadelphia: W.B. Saunders; 1990. Pp. 347–349.
31. Fink A. Analyzing evaluation data. Chapter 7 in *Evaluation Fundamentals,* Pp. 132–154.
32. Norman GR, Streiner DL. *PDQ Statistics.* Toronto: B.C. Decker, 1986. Pp. 1–172.
33. Shott S. *Statistics for Health Professionals.* Philadelphia: W. B. Saunders; 1990. Pp. 1–418.
34. Morris LL, Fitz-Gibbon CT, Freeman ME. *How to Communicate Evaluation Findings* (book number 9). In *Program Evaluation Kit,* Pp. 9–89.

CHAPTER EIGHT

Curriculum Maintenance and Enhancement

THE DYNAMIC NATURE OF CURRICULA

A curriculum that is static gradually declines and dies. A successful curriculum is continually developing. It must respond to evaluation results and feedback, to changes in the knowledge base and the material requiring mastery, to changes in resources (including faculty), to changes in its targeted learners, and to changes in institutional and societal values and needs. A successful curriculum requires *understanding, sustenance,* and *management of change* to maintain its strengths and to promote further improvement. *Related activities,* such as development of the environment in which the curriculum occurs, faculty development, networking with colleagues at other institutions, and scholarly activity, can also strengthen a curriculum.

UNDERSTANDING ONE'S CURRICULUM

To appropriately nurture a curriculum and manage change, one must understand the curriculum and appreciate its complexity—not only the written curriculum but also its learners, its faculty, its support staff, the processes by which it is administered and evaluated, and the setting in which it takes place. Table 8.1 provides a list of the various areas related to a curriculum that are in need of assessment. Table 8.2 lists some meth-

Table 8.1.   Areas for Assessment and Potential Change

The Written or Intended Curriculum

Goals and objectives	Are they understood and accepted by all involved in the curriculum? Are they realistic? Can some be deleted? Should some be altered? Do others need to be added? Are they measurable?
Content	Is the amount just right, too little, or too much? Does the content still match the objectives? Can some content be deleted? Should other content be updated or added?
Curricular materials	Are they being read and used? How useful are the various components perceived to be? Can some be deleted? Should others be altered? Should new materials be added?
Methods	Are they well executed by faculty and well received by learners? Have they been sufficient to achieve curricular objectives? Are additional methods needed to prevent decay of learning?
Congruence	Does the curriculum on paper match the curriculum in reality? If not, is that a problem? Does one or the other need to be changed?

The Environment/Setting of the Curriculum

Space	Is there sufficient space to support the various activities of the curriculum? For clinical curricula, is there sufficient space for learners to see patients? to consult references? to meet with preceptors?
Equipment and supplies	Are there sufficient equipment and supplies to support the curriculum while in progress? to support and reinforce learning after completion of the curriculum? For example: (a) Is there audiovisual equipment to support learning of interviewing skills? (b) Are there sufficient, easily accessible references to support clinical practice experiences? (c) Do the residents' clinical practices have the equipment to support the performance of learned skills and procedures?
Clinical experience	Is there sufficient concentrated clinical experience to support learning during the course of the curriculum? Is there sufficient clinical experience to reinforce learning after completion of the main curriculum? If there is insufficient patient volume or case mix, do alternative clinical experiences need to found or do alternative approaches need to be developed, such as a simulated patient program? Are curricular objectives and general programmatic goals (e.g., efficiency, cost-effectiveness, customer service, record keeping, communication between referring and consulting practitioners, and provision of needed services) supported by clinical practice operations? Do support staff support the curriculum?

Table 8.1.   *(continued)*

Learning climate	Is the climate cooperative or competitive? Are learners encouraged to communicate or to hide what they don't know? Is the curriculum sufficiently learner-centered and -directed? sufficiently teacher-centered and -directed? Are learners encouraged and supported in identifying and pursuing their own learning needs and goals related to the curriculum?
Associated settings	Is learning from the curriculum supported and reinforced in the learners' prior, concomitant, and subsequent settings? If not, is there an opportunity to influence those settings?

Administration of the Curriculum

Scheduling	Are schedules understandable, accurate, realistic, and helpful? Are they put out far enough in advance? Are they adhered to? How are scheduling changes managed?
Preparation and distribution of curricular materials	Is this being accomplished in a timely and consistent manner?
Collection, collation, and distribution of evaluation information	Is this being accomplished in a consistent and timely manner? If there are several different evaluation forms, can they be consolidated into one form or administered at one time, to decrease respondent fatigue?
Communication	Are changes in and important information about the curriculum being communicated to the appropriate individuals in a user-friendly, understandable, and timely manner?

Evaluation

Congruence	Is what is being evaluated consistent with the goals, objectives, content, and methods of the curriculum? Does the evaluation reflect the main priorities of the curriculum?
Response rate	Is it sufficient to be representative of learners, faculty, or others involved in or affected by the curriculum?
Accuracy	Is the information reliable and valid?
Usefulness	Does the evaluation provide timely, easily understandable, and useful information to learners, faculty, curriculum coordinators, and relevant others?

Faculty

Reliability/accessibility	How reliable are the faculty members in performing their curricular responsibilities? Are they devoting more or less time to the curriculum than expected? How accessible are faculty members in responding to learner questions and individual learner needs? Do faculty members schedule free time for discussion before or after sessions?
Teaching/facilitation skills	How skillful are faculty members at assessing the learners' needs, imparting information, asking questions, providing feedback, stimulating self-directed learning, and creating a learning environment that is open, honest, exciting, and fun?

Table 8.1. *(continued)*

Nature of the learner-faculty relationship	Is the relationship more authoritative or collaborative? more teacher-centered or learner-centered? For clinical pre-cepting, does the learner see patients on his or her own? Does the learner observe faculty while faculty are seeing patients or while faculty are assuming other roles? Are learners exposed to faculty members' professional life outside of the curriculum, e.g., clinical practice, research, community work? Do learners get to know faculty members as persons and get to see how faculty balance professional, family, and personal life? Do faculty serve as good role models?
Satisfaction	Do faculty members feel adequately recognized and rewarded for their teaching? Do they feel that their role is an important one? Are they enthusiastic? How satisfied are faculty members with clinical practice, teaching, and their professional lives in general?
Involvement	To what extent are faculty involved in the curriculum? Do faculty complete evaluation forms in a timely manner? Do they attend scheduled meetings? Do they provide useful suggestions for improving the curriculum?
Learners	
Achievement of curriculum objectives	Have cognitive, affective, psychomotor, process, and out-come objectives been achieved? Are learners responsible in meeting their obligations to the curriculum?
Satisfaction	How satisfied are learners with various aspects of the curriculum?
Involvement	To what extent are learners involved in the curriculum? Do they complete evaluation forms in a timely manner? Do they attend scheduled activities and meetings? Do they provide useful suggestions for improving the curriculum?
Application	Do learners apply their learning in other settings and con-texts? Do they teach others what they have learned?

ods of assessing how a curriculum is functioning. *Program evaluation* (discussed in Chapter 7) provides objective and representative subjective feedback on some of these areas. Methods that promote *informal information exchange,* such as site visits, observation of curricular components, and individual or group meetings with learners, faculty, and support staff, can enrich one's understanding of a curriculum. These methods can also build relationships that help to maintain and further develop a curriculum.

EXAMPLE: The General Internal Medicine (GIM) Residency Program at Johns Hopkins Bayview Medical Center has developed a community-based clinical experience for residents in order to expose them to efficiently operating, real-world primary care practices and to foster learning from a broader range of patient problems than is encountered in the hospital-based medical clinic. Teams of four PGY-2 and -3 residents and one faculty leader constitute firms that are assigned to separate community-based practices (CBPs). Residents are assigned every third month to an ambulatory block rotation that includes three sessions per

Table 8.2.   Methods of Assessing How a Curriculum is Functioning

---

Program evaluation (Chapter 7)
Learner/faculty/staff/patient questionnaires
Objective measures of skills and performance
Focus groups of learners, faculty, staff, patients
Other systematically collected data
Regular/periodic meetings with learners, faculty, staff
Special retreats and strategic planning sessions
Site visits
Informal observation of curricular components, learners, faculty, staff
Informal discussions with learners, faculty, staff

---

week at their CBP. Representative feedback on the CBP experience is received yearly from questionnaires completed by firm residents and faculty. Quarterly practice reports provide information on the number of different patients seen, number of patients seen per hour scheduled, fee-for-service revenue generated, billing profiles, and referral patterns. Record keeping and preventive care audits are conducted yearly on all CBP providers. Informal feedback on how the CBP experience is functioning is received at weekly conferences, during which firm residents share experiences with one another and with the residency program director. Monthly, CBP firm leaders and persons from the hospital-based medical clinic meet to share experiences, to identify and address problems, and to plan. Minutes from quarterly meetings of residents with their faculty advisors, twice-yearly dinner meetings of firm residents and faculty, and frequent informal meetings with residents and faculty provide additional information for the program director. Finally, strengths, weaknesses, and future directions for the residency program are brainstormed every three years in a strategic planning meeting that includes residents, CBP, and hospital-based faculty. Through these various and complementary mechanisms, the program director develops a good understanding of the CBP experience.

MANAGEMENT OF CHANGE

Most curricula require midcourse, end-of-cycle, and/or end-of-year changes. Changes may be prompted by informal feedback; by evaluation results; by the evolving needs of learners, faculty, institutions or society; or by changes in available resources. *Before expending resources* to make curricular changes, however, *it is often wise to establish that the need for change (a) is sufficiently important, (b) affects a significant number of people, and (c) will persist if it is not addressed.*

It is also helpful to consider *at what level needs should be addressed and changes made.* Minor operational changes that are necessary for the smooth functioning of a curriculum are most efficiently made at the level of the curriculum coordinator or core group responsible for managing the curriculum. More complicated needs that require in-depth analysis and thoughtful planning for change may best be assigned to a carefully selected task group. Other needs may best be discussed and addressed in meetings of learners, faculty, and/or staff. Before implementing major curricular changes, it is often wise to ensure broad, representative support. It can also be helpful to pilot major or complex changes before implementing them fully.

EXAMPLE: The firm system described above was implemented in July 1994. Previously, GIM residents had been assigned to a four- to six-week CBP block rotation at the beginning of their PGY-2 year. Thereafter, residents spent from no sessions per month to one session per week at their CBP, depending on their hospital rotation. Residents enjoyed their CBP block rotation, but had for years complained of the competing demands they felt between inpatient rotations and their CBP experience subsequent to the block rotation. CBP faculty complained of frequent scheduling changes and loss of a resident's identity with a practice subsequent to the ambulatory block month. At a meeting of GIM residents and faculty in November 1993, the firm system described above was brainstormed and discussed. At this and subsequent meetings, the idea received strong support from CBP faculty and GIM residents, who were willing to give up some elective time to accomplish the change. Approval for the change was obtained from the department chairman. Implementation details were worked out by the GIM Residency Program Director in meetings with the residents, CBP faculty, and Chief Resident who is responsible for resident scheduling.

SUSTAINING THE CURRICULUM TEAM

The curriculum team includes not only the faculty but also the support staff and learners, all of whom are crucial to a curriculum's success. It is, therefore, important to attend to processes that motivate, develop, and support the team. These processes include orientation, communication, involvement, faculty development and team activities, recognition, and celebration (Table 8.3).

EXAMPLE: *Sustaining the Curriculum Team.* The above examples demonstrate how a system of informal, formal, and social meetings can increase the involvement of faculty and residents in program assessment and change.

Previously, medical directors and site administrators had been involved in a strategic planning process that identified primary care education as one of the missions of CBPs.

Teaching contributions constitute one factor that determines a faculty member's distribution in the practices' financial incentive system.

Community-based preceptors can be given faculty appointments and benefits, such as free access to a medical school's Continuing Medical Education (CME) courses or to a university's computer network.

Periodic meetings with office staff can orient the staff to the goals of a clinical practice curriculum, can invite feedback on and suggestions for improving the curriculum, and can develop in the staff a sense of involvement and commitment to the curriculum.

THE LIFE OF A CURRICULUM

A curriculum that does not keep pace with the needs of its learners, its faculty, its institution, its resources, patients, and society does a disservice to its constituents and is likely to deteriorate or die prematurely. One that does keep pace is likely to continually change and improve. After a few years it may differ markedly from its initial form. As health problems and societal needs evolve, even a well-conceived curriculum that has been carefully maintained and developed may appropriately be down-scaled or come to an end.

EXAMPLE: Because of a rapidly changing epidemiology and knowledge base, a successful curriculum on the management of HIV-infected patients is likely to be much different today than it was several years ago. If, in the future, effective preventive measures markedly reduce the prevalence of HIV infection, and simple curative treatment regimens become available for afflicted patients, there may no longer be the need for a separate curriculum on HIV infection.

Table 8.3.   Methods of Motivating, Developing, and Supporting a Curriculum Team

Method	Mechanisms
Orientation and communication	
▪ Goals and objectives	▪ Syllabi/handouts
▪ Guidelines/standards	▪ Meetings
▪ Evaluation results	▪ Memos
▪ Program changes	▪ Newsletters
▪ Rationale for above	
▪ Learner, faculty, staff, patient experiences	
Involvement of faculty, learners, staff	
▪ Goal and objective setting	▪ Questionnaires/interviews
▪ Guideline development	▪ Informal one-on-one meetings
▪ Curricular changes	▪ Group meetings
▪ Determining evaluation and feedback needs	▪ Task group membership
	▪ Strategic planning
Team activities	
	▪ Team teaching/coteaching
	▪ Faculty development activities
	▪ Retreats
	▪ Task groups to analyze/assess needs
	▪ Strategic planning groups
Recognition and celebration	
	▪ Private communication
	▪ Public recognition
	▪ Rewards
	▪ Parties and other social gatherings

RELATED ACTIVITIES THAT CAN STRENGTHEN A CURRICULUM

A curriculum can be strengthened not only by improvements in the existing curriculum per se but also by related activities. These activities include improvements in the setting or environment in which the curriculum takes place, faculty development, communication and sharing across institutions (networking), and relevant scholarly activity. The curriculum coordinator should be aware of how such activities might affect one's curriculum and should support such activities whenever appropriate.

Environmental Development

Changes in the environment in which a curriculum takes place can *create new opportunities* for the curriculum, *reinforce* the learning that has occurred, and *support* its *application by learners.* For example, practice development activities often affect clinical curricula. New institutional or extrainstitutional resources might be used to benefit a curriculum.

EXAMPLE: *Development of Clinical Settings.* An excellent lecture and small-group discussion curriculum on gynecology and women's health for internal medicine residents might be hampered by the lack of sufficient clinical training experiences that focus on the curriculum's goals. The development of a women's health program by an associated institution that concentrates the provision of preventive services for women could improve student and resident training in birth control counseling and management, breast and cervical cancer screening, and osteoporosis prevention—all foci of the curriculum. The development of medical record systems, computerized information systems, and well-trained support staff in the residents' primary care practices that promote and monitor the provision of preventive care services could support the application in real practice of what the residents learn in the curriculum. For the faculty in the same practices, an incentive system that rewards the provision of preventive services could create faculty support for the above changes and could promote the development of role models for residents and students.

EXAMPLE: *New Resources.* Providing all residents with handheld computers so that they can create databases for their clinical experience creates the opportunity for residents to track their clinical experience relevant to that curriculum.

Faculty Development

One of the most important resources for any curriculum is its faculty. As discussed in Chapter 6, a curriculum may benefit from faculty development efforts specifically targeted toward the needs of the curriculum. Institutionwide, regional, or national faculty development programs (see Appendix B) that train faculty in specific content areas, or in time management, teaching, curriculum development, management, or research skills may also benefit a curriculum.

EXAMPLE: Almost all the part-time faculty who serve as ambulatory care preceptors for residents and medical students in the community-based practices associated with the Johns Hopkins Bayview Medical Center participate in the nine-month, one-half-day per-week Teaching Skills portion of the Johns Hopkins Faculty Development Program for Clinician-Educators. This program provides training in time management, feedback, precepting, small-group teaching, communication, lecturing, and management skills.

Networking

Faculty responsible for a curriculum at one institution can benefit from and be invigorated by *communication with colleagues at other institutions* (1). Conceptual clarity and understanding of one's own curriculum is usually enhanced as one prepares it for publication or presentation. New ideas and approaches may come from the comments of those who review one's manuscript or from the interchange that occurs when one presents one's own work to colleagues and hears about or experiences their work. Multi-institutional efforts can produce products, such as annotated bibliographies, articles (2), texts (3–5), and curricula (6–7) that improve upon or transcend the capabilities of faculty at a single institution. The opportunity for such interchange and collaboration can be provided at professional meetings and through professional organizations.

EXAMPLE: There are usually one to a few internal medicine faculty responsible for teaching medical consultation on surgical, obstetric, and psychiatric patients at any single institution. The Medical Consultation Interest Group of the Society of General Internal Medicine has provided the opportunity for such faculty to meet yearly, update medical knowledge, and share curricula and teaching approaches.

EXAMPLE: The American Academy on Physician and Patient sponsors courses, meetings, and interest groups for teachers of interviewing skills and of the psychosocial domain of medical practice that provide opportunities for faculty development, the sharing of curricula and teaching approaches, collaborative work relevant to curricula, and collaborative research (see Appendix B: Additional Resources).

Scholarly Activity

Finally, *scholarly inquiry* can enrich a curriculum by increasing the breadth and depth of knowledge and understanding of its faculty, by creating a sense of excitement among faculty and learners, and by providing the opportunity for learners to engage in scholarly projects. Scholarly activities may include original research or critical reviews in the subject matter of the curriculum or in the methods of teaching and learning that subject matter.

EXAMPLE: *Mentored Scholarly Activity by Learners.* A curriculum in informatics and evidence-based medicine requires that each PGY-1 resident complete and present a critical review of a preventive, diagnostic, or treatment modality of her or his choice at the end of the one-month rotation. This project creates the opportunity for residents and their faculty mentors to apply the critical thinking, clinical decision-making, literature search, and computer slide preparation skills that are emphasized in the curriculum.

EXAMPLE: *Scholarly Activity by Faculty.* Faculty involved in a curriculum development project on domestic violence became interested in the prevalence and clinical characteristics of domestic violence among female primary care patients. The faculty assembled a team to conduct a study (8, 9) that took place in the community-based practices described in previous examples. The faculty received support from an institutional research grant and from the administration of the practices. The expertise and new knowledge that the faculty gained from this study have enriched the domestic violence curriculum, which became integrated into a new gynecology/women's health curriculum.

CONCLUSION

Attending to processes that maintain and enhance a curriculum helps the curriculum remain relevant and vibrant. These processes help a curriculum to evolve in a direction of continuous improvement.

QUESTIONS

For the curriculum you are coordinating, planning, or would like to be planning, please answer the following:

1. As curriculum coordinator, what methods will you use (Table 8.2) to *understand* the curriculum in its complexity (Table 8.1)?

2. How will you implement *minor changes*? *major changes*?

3. What methods (Table 8.3) will you use to maintain the *motivation and involvement* of your faculty? of your support staff?

4. What *related activities* will you encourage or support that could strengthen your curriculum?

GENERAL REFERENCES

Bland CJ, Schmitz CC, Stritter FT, Henry RC, Aluise JJ. *Successful Faculty in Academic Medicine: Essential Skills and How to Acquire Them.* New York: Springer Publishing; 1990.
> This book comprehensively addresses what faculty skills are essential for success in academic medicine and how these skills should be learned. The authors build on the book by McGaghie and Frey (listed below) by describing a model faculty development curriculum that focuses on the five domains of education, administration, research, written communication, and professional academic skills. This book is an excellent resource for faculty development. 315 pages.

Fisher D, Vilas S. *Power Networking: 55 Secrets for Personal and Professional Success.* Austin, Tex.: Mountain Harbor Publications; 1992.
> Reader friendly and useful for those in business or the professions, this book discusses networking, including results and relationships, effectiveness and efficacy, graciousness and persistence. Included are a self-assessment questionnaire and many tips on and examples of how to use networking with others to achieve one's goals. 191 pages.

King JA, Morris LY, Fitz-Gibbon CT. *How to Assess Program Implementation.* Newbury Park, Calif.: Sage Publications; 1987.
> Maintenance and continual improvement of a program involves evaluation. The focus of this book is on planning and executing an evaluation of how well a program has been implemented. The appendix contains over 300 questions for an implementation evaluation of all aspects of a program, which in turn can be used for initial program planning or subsequent program modification. 143 pages.

McGaghie WC, Frey JJ, eds. *Handbook for the Academic Physician.* New York: Springer-Verlag; 1986.
> This multiauthored practical handbook is a source for building a successful career in academic medicine. There are sections on professional development, medical education, clinical research, professional communications, and ethics. 398 pages.

Scholtes PR. *The Team Handbook: How to Use Teams to Improve Quality.* Madison, Wis.: Joiner Associates; 1988.
> This is an easy-to-use manual written for business organizations. It has direct applicability to programs/projects in medical care organizations. Discussed are quality improvement concepts; team decision-making tools; development of an improvement plan; and teamwork principles, activities, and exercises. 302 pages.

Whitman N. Managing faculty development. In Whitman N, Weiss E, Bishop FM, eds., *Executive Skills for Medical Faculty.* Salt Lake City: University of Utah School of Medicine; 1989. Pp. 99–106.
> In this book, managing faculty development to improve teaching skills is discussed as a needed executive function. Five strategies are offered to promote education as a product of the medical school: rewards, assistance, feedback, connoisseurship (developing a taste for good teaching), and creativity.

SPECIFIC REFERENCES

1. Woods SE, Reid A, Arndt JE, Curtis P, Stritter FT. Collegial networking and faculty vitality. *Fam Med* 1997; 29(1):45–49.
2. Williamson PR, Smith R, Kern DE, Lipkin Jr. M, Barker LR, Hoppe RB, Florek J. The medical interview and psychosocial aspects of medicine: block curricula for residents. *J Gen Intern Med* 1992; 7:235–242.
3. Lipkin Jr. ML, Putnam SM, Lazare A, eds. *The Medical Interview: Clinical Care, Education, and Research.* New York: Springer-Verlag; 1995.

4. ACP Governors' Class of 1996. *Learning from Practitioners: Office-Based Teaching of Internal Medicine Residents.* Philadelphia: American College of Physicians; 1995.

5. Deutsch SI, Noble J, eds. *Community-Based Teaching: A Guide to Developing Education Programs for Medical Students and Residents in the Practitioner's Office.* Philadelphia: American College of Physicians; 1997.

6. Goroll AH, Morrison G, Bass EB, Fortin AH, Mumford L. *Core Medicine Clerkship: Curriculum Guide.* Washington, D.C.: Division of Medicine, Bureau of Health Professions, Health Resources and Services Administration, 1995.

7. FCIM (Federated Council of Internal Medicine) Task Force on Internal Medicine Residency Curriculum. *Graduate Education in Internal Medicine: A Resource Guide to Curriculum Development.* Ende J, Kelly M, Ramsey P, Sox H, eds. Philadelphia: American College of Physicians, 1997.

8. McCauley J, Kern DE, Kolodner K, Dill L, Schroeder AF, DeChant HK, Ryden J, Bass EB, Derogatis LR. The "battering syndrome": prevalence and clinical characteristics of domestic violence in primary care internal medicine practices. *Ann Intern Med* 1995; 123:737–746.

9. McCauley J, Kern DE, Kolodner K, Dill L, Schroeder AF, DeChant HK, Ryden J, Derogatis LR, Bass EB. Clinical characteristics of adult female primary care patients with a history of childhood abuse: unhealed wounds. *JAMA* 1997; 277: 1362–1368.

CHAPTER NINE

Dissemination

DEFINITION

Dissemination of a curriculum refers to (a) efforts to promote consideration, adaptation, or adoption of a curriculum by others or (b) the administration of the curriculum to new audiences.

CHOICE OF TARGET AUDIENCE

Dissemination efforts may be targeted at individuals within one's institution, individuals at other institutions, or individuals who are not affiliated with any particular institution. The ideal target audience for dissemination of a curriculum depends on the nature of the curriculum.

EXAMPLE: The ideal audience for disseminating a curriculum for medical students on delivering primary care to an inner-city indigent population might be the faculty and deans of medical schools located in major cities. In contrast, a curriculum on ethical issues in managed care may be worth disseminating more widely, because the targeted learners include health care providers in practice as well as those in training.

WHY BOTHER?

The dissemination of a new or improved curriculum can be important for several reasons. Dissemination can do the following:

- *Help address a health problem:* As indicated in Chapter 2, the ultimate purpose of a curriculum in medical education is to address a problem that affects the health of the public or a given population (1, 2). To maximize the positive effect of a curriculum, it is necessary to share the curriculum with others who are dealing with the same problem.
- *Stimulate change:* An innovative curriculum can create excitement and stimulate change within medical institutions (3).
- *Provide feedback to curriculum developers:* By disseminating a curriculum, developers can obtain valuable feedback from others who may have unique perspectives on the curriculum. This external feedback can promote further development of the curriculum (see Chapter 8).
- *Increase interchange and collaboration:* Dissemination efforts may lead to increased interchange of ideas between people within an institution or in different institutions who are interested in the same issues. Such interchange may lead to active collaboration. The resulting teamwork is likely to lead to development of an even better curriculum or to other products that would not have been developed by individuals working separately.
- *Prevent redundant work:* Other persons may be struggling with the same issues that require curriculum development and evaluation. By disseminating a curriculum, developers can minimize the extent to which different people expend time and energy repeating work that has been done elsewhere. Instead, developers can devote their time and energy to building upon what has already been accomplished.
- *Help curriculum developers achieve recognition and academic advancement:* Medical school faculty may devote a substantial amount of time to the development of curricula but may have difficulties achieving academic advancement if this portion of their overall work is not recognized as representing significant scholarship. One important criterion for judging the significance of scholarly work is the degree to which the work has had an effect at a local, regional, national, or international level. For curriculum developers who are working in an academic setting, successful dissemination of curriculum work has considerable value because it demonstrates that the work has had a broad influence. Medical school promotion committees are beginning to recognize the value of this type of work and will increasingly look for evidence that curriculum work has been effectively disseminated (4, 5).

EXAMPLE: *Benefits of Dissemination.* An innovative curriculum for internal medicine residents on interviewing skills and the psychosocial domain of medical practice was developed by faculty at the Johns Hopkins Bayview Medical Center. Dissemination of this and related curricula has occurred in workshops and in published articles (6–8). This dissemination has been of value to faculty at other institutions who were independently working on ways to enhance clinical training in this area. It has generated feedback and promoted interactions and discussions that have led to improvements in the original curriculum. It has led to collaborative work that resulted in an additional publication (9). As a result of the successful dissemination of the curriculum, the curriculum developers have gained national recognition for their work. This recognition has been cited as an important achievement when the responsible faculty members have been reviewed and approved for promotion by the medical school's promotion and tenure committee.

Are dissemination efforts worth the time and effort required? In many cases, the answer is yes, even for individuals who do not need academic advancement. If the curriculum developer performed an appropriate problem identification and general needs assessment, as discussed in Chapter 2, the curriculum will likely address an important problem that has not been adequately addressed previously. If this is the case, the curriculum is likely to be of value to others. The challenge is to decide how the curriculum should be disseminated and how much time and effort the curriculum developer can realistically devote to dissemination efforts. The final decision usually will involve a trade-off between the degree of dissemination desired and the amount of time that the curriculum developer can afford to spend on dissemination.

WHAT SHOULD BE DISSEMINATED?

The first decision to make when developing plans for disseminating curriculum work is to *determine whether the entire curriculum or any parts of it should be disseminated.* The curriculum developer can refer to the problem identification and general needs assessment to determine the extent of the need for the curriculum and to determine whether the curriculum truly represents a new contribution to the field. The results of the evaluation of a curriculum will also help determine whether any aspect of the curriculum is worth disseminating.

In some cases, dissemination efforts will focus on promoting adoption of a *complete curriculum* by other sites. Usually, this approach requires some allowance for modifications to meet the unique needs of the learners at these sites.

EXAMPLE: *Complete Curriculum.* Members of the Society of General Internal Medicine and the Clerkship Directors in Internal Medicine, under a contract from the federal Health Resources and Services Administration (HRSA), designed a curriculum for the core clerkship in internal medicine. To disseminate the work, a curriculum guide was prepared that described the need for the curriculum, specific learner objectives, proposed educational strategies, and methods of evaluation (10). This guide was published by HRSA and distributed to internal medicine clerkship directors in all U.S. medical schools. The work also was disseminated through presentations at meetings of the American Association of Medical Colleges, the Clerkship Directors in Internal Medicine, and the Society of General Internal Medicine.

EXAMPLE: *Complete Curriculum.* The Task Force on Internal Medicine Residency Curriculum of the Federated Council of Internal Medicine (FCIM) led an effort that united all the major internal medicine organizations and that solicited nationally representative input to define the essentials of an internal medicine residency training program. The task force has published its results as a resource guide for curriculum development for internal medicine residencies (11, 12). The guide provides nationally developed consensus recommendations on learning domains, prioritized learner objectives, and learning content. It also identifies the facilities, faculty roles, team structure, educational methods, and evaluation systems that can facilitate the accomplishment of learning. It discusses current challenges in terms of new curriculum development. The resource guide provides a nationally derived, consensus-based core that identifies what all residents should learn, while deferring to local faculty with regard to how, where, and when that learning should take place.

In other cases, it is appropriate to limit dissemination efforts to *specific products of the curriculum development process* that are likely to be of value to others. The problem identification and general needs assessment (Step 1) may yield new insights about a problem, which may warrant dissemination. Such insights and justification for dissemination may occur when a comprehensive review of the literature on a topic has been performed, or when a systematic survey on the extent of a problem has been conducted. The needs assessment of targeted learners (Step 2) may yield unique insights about the need for a curriculum and would merit dissemination if the targeted learners are reasonably representative of other potential learners. When such insights and justification for dissemination occur, the methods employed in the needs assessment will need to be carefully described so that other groups can determine whether the results of the needs assessment are valid and applicable to them. In some cases, the formulation of learning objectives for a topic (Step 3) may, by itself, represent an important contribution to a field, thereby calling for some degree of dissemination. In other cases, it may be worthwhile to focus the dissemination efforts on specific methods for implementing a curriculum (Step 4). Most often, however, the results of the evaluation of a curriculum (Step 6) are the focus of dissemination efforts because people are more likely to adopt an innovative approach, or to abandon a traditional approach, when there is evidence regarding the efficacy, or lack of efficacy, of the approach.

> **EXAMPLE:** *Step 1.* As part of the *problem identification and general needs assessment* for designing a new curriculum for the medical school core clerkship in internal medicine, a clerkship director performed a review of the published literature on nontraditional approaches to the internal medicine clerkship. This literature review was disseminated in a targeted manner by submitting a report to the U.S. Health Resources and Services Administration (HRSA) (13). HRSA used this report to help develop strategies for promoting changes in medical school training that will better prepare students for careers in a changing health care environment.

> **EXAMPLE:** *Step 2.* As part of the *needs assessment of targeted learners* for a curriculum on practice guidelines for internists, a group performed a survey of internists to assess their familiarity with, confidence in, and attitudes toward practice guidelines. The results of this survey were published in a leading medical journal (14).

> **EXAMPLE:** Step 3. Faculty at the University of Wisconsin led an effort to define learning *objectives* for an internal medicine residency curriculum. The resulting comprehensive list of learning objectives was published (15).

> **EXAMPLE:** *Step 4.* A team of gynecologists and internists designed a curriculum on office gynecology for the practicing internist. *Educational strategies* were developed for teaching internists about specific common gynecologic problems encountered in medical practice. This curriculum has been disseminated through *workshops and courses* that have been presented at national meetings of the Society of General Internal Medicine. The content of the curriculum also is being disseminated by incorporating curriculum material into a new *textbook* on gynecology for the internist.

> **EXAMPLE:** *Step 6.* A team of family practitioners designed an educational program to reduce unnecessary laboratory tests by residents. An *evaluation* of the success of this program was disseminated through publication in a peer-reviewed medical journal (16).

Table 9.1.   Modes of Disseminating Curriculum Work

- Presentations of abstracts, workshops, or courses to individuals and groups within specific institutions
- Presentations of abstracts, workshops, or courses at regional, national, and international professional meetings
- Creation of a multi-institutional interest group
- Submission of curricular materials to an educational clearinghouse
- Use of computerized communication systems (e.g., World Wide Web)
- Preparation and distribution of instructional videotapes or audiotapes
- Creation and distribution of instructional computer software
- Publication of an article in a professional journal
- Publication of a manual, book, or book chapter

HOW SHOULD CURRICULUM WORK BE DISSEMINATED?

To most effectively disseminate a curriculum, it is important to develop a coherent strategy. Developing such a strategy requires an explicit delineation of the purpose of and target audience for the dissemination efforts. A realistic assessment of the time and resources available for dissemination is necessary to ensure that the dissemination strategy is feasible. Once the purpose of the dissemination has been defined and available resources identified, the curriculum developer must choose the most appropriate modes of dissemination (see Table 9.1 and text below). Ideally, the curriculum developer will use a variety of dissemination modes to maximize the effectiveness of the dissemination effort.

Presentations

Usually, the first mode of dissemination involves *written or oral presentations to key people within the setting where the curriculum was developed.* These presentations may be targeted at potential learners or at faculty who will need to be involved in the curriculum. The presentations may also be directed at leaders who can provide important support or resources for the curriculum.

Once a curriculum has been established within the setting of its origin, dissemination to *other sites* is appropriate. An efficient way to disseminate a new or improved curriculum to other sites is to present the curriculum work at regional, national, or international *meetings of professional societies* that include clinicians, teachers, and educators. A workshop or minicourse is an appropriate format for presenting the content or methods of a curriculum. A presentation that follows a research abstract format is appropriate for presenting results of a needs assessment or a curriculum evaluation. Guidelines have been published for research presentations (17). As illustrated in Table 9.2, information from the six-step curriculum development cycle can fit nicely into the format for an abstract presentation.

Multi-institutional Interest Groups

In some cases, presentation of curriculum work at professional meetings may stimulate interest in creating a multi-institutional interest group. Once such a group is created, communication between members of the group may occur in a number of ways, such as in-person meetings, telephone contact, or E-mail.

Educational Clearinghouses

To disseminate curriculum work even more widely, written curriculum materials can be submitted to an educational clearinghouse, which may or may not be computerized (see Appendix B: Additional Resources). This mode of dissemination is particularly appropriate for disseminating the curricular objectives and syllabus materials, but also may be useful for disseminating instruments used in the needs assessment and/or curriculum evaluation. Information about the existence of an educational clearinghouse for a particular clinical domain generally can be obtained from the professional societies that have a vested interest in educational activities in that domain.

Computerized Communication Systems

The recent emergence of computerized communication systems, such as the Internet, provides a tremendous opportunity for curriculum developers to share curricular materials with anyone who has access to a computer system (18). To take advantage of this potential mode of dissemination, technical support and computer training are needed.

Instructional Videotapes or Audiotapes

Another way to disseminate teaching methods and curriculum content to other sites is to prepare a video- or audiotape of curriculum components. The availability of the video- or audiotape can be advertised through an educational clearinghouse or through any computerized information system.

Instructional Computer Software

Curriculum developers with a high degree of computer expertise can create computer software for a curriculum. The software can be interactive and menu driven, which can make a learning program very learner-centered. Such software can be advertised through the same types of channels mentioned above.

Publication

One of the most traditional, but still underutilized, modes of disseminating medical education work is publication in a *medical journal or textbook*. When a curriculum developer seeks to disseminate a comprehensive curriculum, it may be wise to consider preparation of a book or manual. On the other hand, the format for original research articles can be used to present results of a needs assessment or a curriculum evaluation (Table 9.2). The format for review articles or meta-analysis can be used to present results of a problem identification and general needs assessment. An editorial or special article format sometimes can be used for other types of work, such as discussion of the most appropriate learning objectives or methods for a needed curriculum.

Many journals will consider articles derived from curriculum work. The curriculum developer will have the best chance of having an article accepted by a journal if the results of the curriculum work are relevant to the majority of the readers of a journal and if

Table 9.2.   Format for an Abstract Presentation or a Curriculum Description/Evaluation Article

I. Introduction
    A. Rationale
        1. Problem identification
        2. General needs assessment
        3. Needs assessment of targeted learners
    B. Purpose
        1. Goals of curriculum
        2. Goals of evaluation: Evaluation questions

II. Materials and methods
    A. Setting
    B. Subjects/power analysis if any
    C. Educational intervention
        1. Relevant specific measurable objectives
        2. Relevant educational strategies
        (3. Resources: Faculty, other personnel, equipment/facilities, costs)*
        (4. Display or offer of educational materials)
    D. Evaluation methods
        1. Evaluation design
        2. Evaluation instruments
            a) Reliability measures if any
            b) Validity measures if any
            c) Display (or offer) of evaluation instruments
        3. Data collection and analysis

III. Results
    A. Data: Tables, figures, graphs, etc.
    B. Statistical analysis

IV. Conclusions and discussion
    A. Summary and discussion of findings
    (B. Comparison to work of others)
    C. Strengths and limitations of work
    D. Conclusions (future directions)

*Items in parentheses are usually omitted from presentations.

that journal has a track record of publishing medical education articles. Curriculum evaluations will most likely be accepted for publication by peer-reviewed journals if such evaluations satisfy common standards of methodology rigor. Table 9.3 displays criteria that may be considered by reviewers of an original article about a curriculum. Even published curricular articles seldom satisfy all of these criteria. Nevertheless, the criteria can serve as a guide to curriculum developers who are interested in publishing their work. Methodologic criteria for controlled trials (19–21), review articles (22–24), and meta-analyses (25, 26) have been published elsewhere.

Diffusion of Innovations

In attempting to disseminate all or parts of a curriculum, it is worthwhile to review what is known about the diffusion of innovations. Factors that promote the likelihood and rapidity of adoption of an innovation include: (a) *relative advantage*—the degree to which an innovation is perceived as superior to existing practice; (b) *compatibility*—the degree to which an innovation is perceived by the adopter as similar to previous experience, beliefs, and values; (c) *simplicity*—the degree to which a new idea is perceived as relatively easy to understand and implement; (d) *trialability*—the degree to which an innovation can be divided into steps and tried out by the adopter; and (e) *observability*—the degree to which the innovation can be seen and appreciated by others (27, 28).

According to the conceptual model described by Rogers (27, 28), individuals pass through *several stages* when deciding whether to adopt an innovative idea. These stages included: (a) *acquisition of knowledge* about an innovation, (b) *persuasion* that the innovation is worth considering, (c) a *decision* to adopt the innovation, (d) *implementation* of the innovation, and (e) *confirmation* that the innovation is worth continuing.

One of the main implications of Rogers's model is that efforts to disseminate an innovative curriculum should involve more than just communication of knowledge about the curriculum. The dissemination strategy should include efforts to *persuade* individuals of the need to consider the curriculum innovation. Efforts at persuasion are best directed at individuals who are most likely to make decisions about implementation of a curriculum or who are most likely to influence other individuals' attitudes or behavior regarding implementation of a curricular innovation. The dissemination strategy also should include efforts to identify barriers (29) to curricular transfer and to *support* those individuals who decide to implement the curriculum. Such efforts usually require direct interpersonal communication, through professional meetings, telephone conversations, or E-mail. In some cases, a site visit may be necessary to achieve optimal communication. Regardless of the mode of communication, it usually is best to identify in a targeted institution a specific individual who will lead the effort to transfer an innovative curriculum to that institution.

Ideally, a collaborative relationship will develop between the original curriculum developer and the adopting group. A *collaborative approach is ideal* because most curricula require modifications when transferred to other settings. Moreover, the establishment of an ongoing collaborative relationship generally strengthens the curriculum for all users and stimulates further innovation and products.

WHAT RESOURCES ARE REQUIRED

To ensure a successful dissemination effort, it is important for the curriculum developer to identify the resources that are required. While the dissemination of curricular work can result in significant benefits to both curriculum developers and others, it is also necessary for the curriculum developer to ensure that the use of limited resources is appropriately balanced among competing needs.

Time and Effort

Disseminating curricular work almost always requires considerable time and effort of the *person or persons responsible.* Unless one is quite experienced in disseminating

Table 9.3.   Criteria That May Be Considered in the Review of an Original Article on a Curriculum

Rationale
- Is there a well reasoned need for the curriculum? (problem identification and general needs assessment)

Setting
- Is the setting clearly described?
- Is the setting sufficiently representative to make the article of interest to readers? (external validity)

Subjects
- Are the learners clearly described? (Specific profession and specialty within profession; educational level, e.g., third-year medical students, PGY-2 residents, or practitioners; needs assessment of targeted learners; sociodemographic information)
- Are the learners sufficiently representative to make the article of interest to readers? (external validity)

Educational intervention
- Are the relevant objectives clearly expressed?
- Are the objectives meaningful and congruent with the rationale for the curriculum?
- Are the educational content and methods described in sufficient detail to be replicated? (If written description is incomplete, are educational materials offered?)
- Are the required resources adequately described (e.g., faculty, faculty development, equipment)?

Evaluation Methods
- Are the methods described in sufficient detail so that the evaluation is replicable?
- Is the evaluation question clear? Are independent and dependent variables clearly defined?
- Are the dependent variables meaningful and congruent with the rationale of the curriculum? (E.g., Is performance measured instead of competence, skill instead of knowledge, when those are the desired or most meaningful effects?)
- Are long-term as well as short-term effects measured?
- Is the evaluation design clear and sufficiently strong to answer the evaluation question?
- Has a power analysis been conducted to determine the likelihood that the evaluation would detect an effect of the desired magnitude?
- Are raters blinded to the status of learners? have inter- and intrarater reliability been assessed?
- Are the measurement instruments described or displayed in sufficient detail? (If incompletely described or displayed, are they offered or referenced?)
- Do the measurement instruments seem to possess face validity? Are they congruent with the evaluation question?
- Have the reliability and validity of the measurement instruments been assessed? Are the reliability and validity sufficient to ensure the accuracy of the measured instruments? Have the measurement instruments been used elsewhere? Have they attained a level of general acceptance? (Rarely are the last two criteria satisfied.)
- Are the statistical methods (parametric vs. nonparametric) appropriate for the type of data collected (nominal, ordinal, numerical; normally distributed vs. skewed; very small vs. larger sample size)? Are the specific statistical tests appropriate to answer the

evaluation question? Have potentially confounding independent variables been controlled for by random allocation or the appropriate statistical methods?
- Are the evaluation methods, as a whole, sufficiently rigorous to ensure the internal validity of the evaluation?

Results
- Is the response rate adequate?
- Are the results of sufficient interest to be worthy of publication? (The paper's introduction and discussion can help address this question.)

Conclusions
- Are the conclusions justified based upon the methodology of the study or report?
- Are the strengths and limitations of the methodology acknowledged?
- Is the paper's contribution to the existing knowledge base clearly and accurately described?

---

curricular work, it is wise to multiply one's initial estimates by a factor of 2 to 4, which is likely to be closer to reality than the original estimate. The least time and effort are required by submissions of already developed curricular products to an educational clearinghouse or web site. More time and effort is required for presentations of abstracts, workshops, and courses, or for the creation of instructional tapes or computer software. Publications generally require the most time and effort. It is also useful to think about the time and effort that will be required of the *recipients* of one's dissemination efforts, and about how that time and effort can be secured and respected.

Personnel

The creation of instructional audiovisual tapes or computer software may require the involvement of *individuals with appropriate technical expertise*. Collaborative approaches with *colleagues* permits the sharing of workload, can help group members maintain interest and momentum, and can provide the type of creative, critical, and supportive interactions that result in a better product than would have been achieved by a single individual. The identification of a *mentor* can be very helpful to individuals who have little experience in disseminating curricular work.

Equipment/Facilities

Equipment needs for dissemination are generally minimal and usually consist of equipment, such as audiovisual equipment or a personal computer, that is already accessible to health professional faculty. Occasionally, software programs may need to be purchased. *Facilities or space* for presentations is usually provided by the recipients. Occasionally a studio may be required for the development of audiovisual tapes.

Funds

Faculty may need to have time protected from other responsibilities in order to accomplish a dissemination effort. Sometimes a faculty member's institution can provide this. Sometimes external funding can provide partial *salary support* (see also Chapter 6 and Appendix B). Funds may also be required for the purchase of necessary new *equipment* or the rental of *facilities*.

CONCLUSIONS

The dissemination of a new or improved curriculum can be valuable to the curriculum developer and curriculum, as well as to others. To be effective in disseminating a curriculum, or the products of a curriculum development process, the curriculum developer must develop a coherent strategy that determines what is worth disseminating, that employs appropriate modes of dissemination, and that makes the best use of available time and resources.

QUESTIONS

For a curriculum that you are coordinating, planning, or would like to be planning, please answer the following:

1. What are the *reasons* that you might want to disseminate part or all of your work?

2. *Which* steps in your curriculum development process would you expect to lead to a discrete *product* worth disseminating to other individuals and groups?

3. Describe a *dissemination strategy* that would fulfill your reasons for wanting to disseminate part or all of your work. Usually this requires more than one mode of dissemination (see Table 9.1).

4. *Estimate the resources, in terms of time and effort, personnel, equipment/facilities and costs* that would be required to implement your dissemination strategy. Is the strategy feasible? Would you need to identify mentors or colleagues to help you develop or execute the dissemination strategy? Multiply your estimate of needed time and effort by a factor of 2 to 4 (which is likely to be closer to reality). Would your plans for dissemination need to be altered or abandoned? Imagine the pleasures and rewards of a successful dissemination effort. Could you afford to abandon your goals for dissemination?

GENERAL REFERENCES

Bauman LJ, Stein REK, Ireys HT. Reinventing fidelity: the transfer of social technology among settings. *Am J of Community Psychology* 1991; 19:619–639.

This article contains a thoughtful discussion of barriers to program diffusion and guidance as to how to implement a program in different sites with different personnel and client populations.

Orlandi MA, Landers C, Weston R, Haley N. Diffusion of Health Promotion Innovations. Chapter 13 in Glanz K, Lewis FM, Rimer BK, eds., *Health Behavior and Health Education.* San Francisco: Jossey-Bass; 1990. Pp. 288–313.

This chapter discusses various aspects of diffusion theory that have direct applicability to the process of translating new health-related research findings or effective interventions into widespread behavior change for the good of society. In doing so, the chapter focuses on three key areas: it reviews the concept of a generic diffusion system and notes some limitations of the classic diffusion model; it describes an alternative research framework that enhances standard approaches to both innovation development and diffusion planning by increasing target group participation; and the chapter provides an example of this research framework in the form of a community-based health promotion study.

Peters R, Sikorski R. Navigating to knowledge: Tools for finding information on the Internet. *JAMA* 1997; 277(6):505–506.

> This short article explores the fundamentals of searching for information on the Internet, especially the World Wide Web, by way of various search engines. To better understand these tools, the article explains how to search for documents, for messages, and for people (telephone numbers, addresses, E-mail).

Rogers EM. *Diffusion of Innovations.* New York: Free Press; 1983.

> This classic text presents a useful framework for understanding how new ideas are communicated to members of a social system. 453 pages.

Westberg J, Jason H. *Making Presentations: Guidebook for Health Professions Teachers.* Boulder, Co.: Center for Instructional Support, Johnson Printing; 1991.

> This is a user-friendly resource for health professionals on all aspects of preparing and giving presentations; stage fright; audiovisuals; and strategies to enhance presentations. 89 pages.

SPECIFIC REFERENCES

1. Golden AS. A model for curriculum development linking curriculum with health needs. In Golden AS, Carlson DG, Hogan JL, eds. *The Art of Teaching Primary Care.* Springer Series on Medical Education, vol. 3. New York: Springer Publishing; 1982. Pp. 9–25.
2. Harden RM. Ten questions to ask when planning a course or curriculum. *Med Educ* 1986; 20:356–365.
3. Sharf BF, Freeman J, Benson J, Rogers J. Organizational rascals in medical education: mid-level innovation through faculty development. *Teaching and Learning in Medicine* 1989; 1:215–220.
4. Lubitz RM. Guidelines for the promotion of clinician-teachers. *J Gen Intern Med* 1997; 12(suppl. 2): S71–S78.
5. Beasley BW, Wright SM, Cofrancesco J, Babbott SF, Thomas PA, Bass EB. Promotion criteria for clinician-educators in the United States and Canada. A survey of promotion committee chairpersons. *JAMA* 1997; 278:723–728.
6. Kern DE, Grayson M, Barker LR, Roca RP, Cole KA, Roter D, Golden AS. Residency training in interviewing skills and the psychosocial domain of medical practice. *J Gen Intern Med* 1989; 4:421–431.
7. Roter DL, Cole KA, Kern DE, Barker LR, Grayson MA. An evaluation of residency training in interviewing skills and the psychosocial domain of medical practice. *J Gen Intern Med* 1990; 5:347–354.
8. Roter DL, Hall JA, Kern DE, Barker LR, Cole KA, Roca RP. Improving physicians' interviewing skills and reducing patients' emotional distress: A randomized clinical trial. *Arch Intern Med* 1995; 155:1877–1884.
9. Williamson PW, Smith R, Kern DE, Lipkin Jr. ML, Barker LR, Hoppe R, Florek J. The medical interview and psychosocial aspects of medicine: Residency block curricula. *J Gen Intern Med* 1992; 7:235–242.
10. Goroll AH, Morrison G, Project Co-Directors. *Core Medicine Clerkship: Curriculum Guide.* Washington, D.C.: Division of Medicine, Bureau of Health Professions, Health Resources and Services Administration, 1995.
11. Ende J, Kelley M, Sox H. The Federated Council of Internal Medicine's resource guide for residency education: An instrument for curricular change. *Ann Intern Med* 1997; 127:454–457.
12. FCIM (Federated Council of Internal Medicine) Task Force on Internal Medicine Residency Curriculum. *Graduate Education in Internal Medicine: A Resource Guide to Curriculum Development.* Ende J, Kelly M, Ramsey P, Sox H, eds. Philadelphia: American College of Physicians; 1997.

13. Mumford LM. A review and analysis of the literature about the non-traditional required internal medicine clerkship, submitted to the Bureau of Health Professions, Health Resources and Services Administration, Department of Health and Human Services, under Contract # 240-93-0029, December 1, 1993. Pp. 1–38.
14. Tunis SR, Hayward RSA, Wilson MC, Rubin HR, Bass EB, Johnston M, Steinberg EP. Internists' attitudes about clinical practice guidelines. *Ann Intern Med* 1994; 120:956–963.
15. Jensen NM, Dirkx JM, editors. *Training for the practice of medicine: A guide for internal medicine residency.* Philadelphia: American College of Physicians; 1989.
16. Dowling PT, Alfonsi G, Brown MI, Culpepper L. An education program to reduce unnecessary laboratory tests by residents. *Acad Med* 1989; 64:410–412.
17. Garson A, Gutgesell HP, Pinsky WW, McNamara DG. The 10-minute talk: Organization, slides, writing and delivery. *Amer Heart J* 1986; 111(1):193–203.
18. Kleeberg P, Masys DR. Telecommunications. In Osheroff JA, ed., *Computers in Clinical Practice: Managing Patients, Information, and Communication.* Philadelphia: American College of Physicians; 1995. Pp. 127–148.
19. Begg C, Cho M, Eastwood S, Horton R, Moher D, Olkin I et al. Improving the quality of reporting of randomized controlled trials: The CONSORT statement. *JAMA* 1996; 276:637–639.
20. The Standards of Reporting Trials Group. A proposal for structured reporting of randomized controlled trials. *JAMA* 1994; 272:1926–1931.
21. The Asilomar Working Group on Recommendations for Reporting of Clinical Trials in the Biomedical Literature. Checklist of information for inclusion in reports of clinical trials. *Ann Intern Med* 1996; 124:741–743.
22. Oxman AD, Guyatt GH. Guidelines for reading literature reviews. *Canadian Med Association J* 1988; 138:697–703.
23. Mulrow CD. The medical review article: State of the science. *Ann Intern Med* 1987; 106:485–488.
24. Haynes RB, Sackett DL, Tugwell P. Problems in handling of clinical and research evidence by medical practitioners. *Arch Intern Med* 1983; 143:1971–1975.
25. Sacks HS, Berrier J, Reitman D, Ancona-Berk VA, Chalmers TC. Meta-analysis of randomized controlled trials. *N Engl J Med* 1987; 316:450–455.
26. Cook DJ, Sackett DL, Spitzer WO. Methodologic guidelines for systematic reviews of randomized control trials in health care from the Potsdam consultation meta-analysis. *J Clin Epidemiol* 1995; 48:167–171.
27. Rogers EM. *Diffusion of Innovations.* New York: Free Press; 1983. Pp. 34–37.
28. Rogers EM. Lessons for guidelines from the diffusion of innovations. *J Quality Improvement* 1995; 21:324–328.
29. Bauman LJ, Stein REK, Ireys HT. Reinventing fidelity: the transfer of social technology among settings. *Am J of Community Psychology* 1991; 19:631–635.

APPENDIX A

Example Curricula

This appendix provides three examples of curricula that have progressed through all 6 steps of curriculum development. The reader may want to review one or more of these examples to see how the various steps of the curriculum development process can relate to one another and be integrated into a whole.

The curricula were chosen to demonstrate differences in focus, scope, and longevity. Two curricula focus on training in limited domains where content can be largely controlled (gynecology and interviewing skills/psychosocial medicine); one curriculum is designed for a clinical training experience in an entire field of medicine where content is largely driven by patient–trainee interactions (ambulatory medical student clerkship). One curriculum was developed during the past one to two years (ambulatory clerkship); another was developed over the past few years (gynecology); and the third has been in existence for over a decade (interviewing skills/psychosocial medicine). Two curricula have progressed to the stage of dissemination (gynecology and interviewing skills/psychosocial medicine).

PRIMARY CARE GYNECOLOGY FOR INTERNAL MEDICINE RESIDENTS

This curriculum was developed in 1993–1994 as part of the curriculum development arm of the Johns Hopkins Faculty Development Program for Clinician Educators. It was implemented during the 1994–1995 academic year as part of the General Internal Medicine (GIM) Residency Program based at Johns Hopkins Bayview Medical Center (JHBMC). Faculty who collaborated in its development included three internists (Richard H. Baker, M.D.; Jeannie McCauley, M.D.; and Janice Ryden, M.D.), one of whom was a medical education fellow at the time, and two gynecologists (Jessica Bienstock, M.D., and Vanessa Cullins, M.D.), one of whom was a gynecology–public health fellow at the time.

Step 1: Problem Identification and General Needs Assessment

Because a literature search revealed only a few relevant references, the curriculum developers also conducted informal interviews with a number of primary care internists, gynecologists, and internal medical residents. The results of the interviews and literature search are summarized in the following table.

Problem Identification	Women's health issues are common in medical practice. A general medical examination or health maintenance visit is a frequent reason for visits to internists. Sixty percent of internists' patients are women. Breast and cervical cancer screening are important components of preventive care. Hormone replacement therapy is an important consideration in postmenopausal women. Other women's health issues that are commonly encountered in primary care practice include domestic violence, vaginal infections/sexually transmitted diseases, use of medications during pregnancy, family planning/birth control, premenstrual syndrome, amenorrhea, dysfunctional uterine bleeding, gynecologic emergencies.
	Internists have been poorly trained to meet many of the women's health needs of their patients.
	Gynecologists have been poorly trained to provide nongynecologic care to female patients.
	A result is that many women receive fragmented, noncomprehensive health care.
	Women's health care may also be inefficient in that some care is duplicated, routine care often requires visits to two separate physicians, and surgically trained gynecologists may spend much time providing routine/preventive care and less time performing higher-level consultations and surgery.
Current Approach	*Society:* There is pressure from third-party payers to provide care efficiently and to limit unnecessary referrals. There is increasing public pressure on health care providers to address the health care needs of women.
	Patients: They may fail to be screened appropriately for early detection of disease. Patients who identify the gynecologist as a primary care physician may fail to seek other general medical preventive interventions, such as cardiac risk factor modification. Internists' referrals can cause fragmentation of care and additional time lost from work. Patients may prefer to see a female health care provider or gynecologist for gynecologic care.
	Physicians: Internists report lack of knowledge, skills, and training in this area; they frequently fail to provide routine gynecologic care to their patients; they frequently refer patients for routine gynecologic care; some may not perceive the provision of routine gynecologic care as their role.
	Medical Educators: Internal medicine residents, for the most part, receive little to no training in women's health/gynecology. Some residencies have developed women's health curricula and/or provide residents with experience in women's health outpatient clinics. Rather than gynecological topics, the emphasis tends to be in-

ternal medicine problems as experienced by women, such as primary prevention of cardiovascular disease in women.

Ideal Approach	*General Internists:* They should know how to do the following:

General Internists: They should know how to do the following:

- Perform breast and pelvic examinations and provide women's preventive care with confidence and competence;
- Manage women's health problems that are common in primary care practice, recognizing that whether specific problems are managed by the primary care physician or gynecologist may vary depending on setting (e.g., rural vs. urban);
- Recognize and initially manage gynecologic emergencies;
- Refer appropriately to gynecologic specialists, recognizing that the indications for referral may vary depending on setting.

Medical Educators: They should provide internal medicine residents with an education that does the following:

- Addresses biases, attitudes, and beliefs of residents with respect to the role of the internist
- Instructs residents in the performance of breast and pelvic examinations by using simulated models and real patients, with observation by and feedback from supervisors
- Ensures that the structure of the residents' continuity practice promotes the provision of routine gynecologic care
- Provides training in the appropriate provision of women's preventive care
- Provides training in the recognition, diagnosis, and management of women's health problems that are common in primary care practice
- Exposes residents to internists who are knowledgeable in primary care gynecology and women's health and who can serve as teachers and role models.

Step 2: Needs Assessment of Targeted Learners

To assess the learning needs of the residents in the JHBMC program, three methods were chosen: (a) questionnaire of all internal medicine residents, (b) chart audit of all internal medicine residents in their hospital-based ambulatory Medical House Staff Practice (MHSP), and (c) informal discussion with selected internal medicine residents and faculty.

Targeted Learners	*PGY-2 (Postgraduate Year 2) and PGY-3 GIM Residents:* Based upon demands from GIM residents and the GIM Program Director, the career path of GIM residents, the availability of curricular time, and the results of the targeted needs assessment, it was decided that the curriculum should be integrated into the ambulatory block rotations of all GIM track residents. Over 90% of GIM track residents pursue generalist careers. Most traditional track residents (over 75%) pursue subspecialty training; they would be able to take the curriculum, if they chose, during elective rotations.

Needs Assessment

Survey Results (November 1993; PGY-1, -2 and -3 GIM Residents):

- Number of pelvics/Paps: Mean was 11/4 for all residents; 17/6 for GIM residents; range 0–100/0–20. Results were probably influenced by the relative inexperience of "first semester" PGY-1 residents, and mean was influenced by an "outlier" resident who performed many pelvic examinations despite barriers.
- Location of pelvic examinations: Emergency room was primary site for experience; community-based practice was a close second for GIM residents; hospital-based MHSP was second for all residents.
- Barriers to providing gynecologic care in MSHP: Lack of time, lack of support from clinic staff, and poor facilities were seen as the major barriers by all residents; all residents tended to disagree with assertions that they will not have to do gynecologic examinations in the future and that gynecologists should do gynecologic examinations rather than internists, GIM residents disagreed more strongly.
- Anticipated future need: GIM residents, on average, predicted that, in the future, they would have to do gynecologic examinations "occasionally" to "frequently"; all residents predicted that they would have to do such examinations "rarely" to "occasionally."
- Desire for gynecologic curriculum: GIM residents "definitely," all residents "probably," wanted a gynecology curriculum. GIM residents preferred two weeks; all residents one week.
- Desired content: Topics in order of preference for GIM residents were hormone replacement, abnormal vaginal bleeding, pelvic and Pap examinations, contraception, sexually transmitted diseases and vaginitis, gynecologic emergencies, domestic violence, pelvic pain, amenorrhea, recurrent urinary tract infections, medications in pregnancy, endometriosis, breast examinations and breast cancer, gynecologic cancers, preconception counseling, premenstrual tension, rape, gynecology in the HIV-positive patient, gynecologic endocrinology. Analysis by all residents was similar, except that all residents rated medications in pregnancy several places higher.

Audit Results:

- 82% of eligible women under age 50 had received a Pap smear: 87.5% were done in gynecology clinic. Only 12.5% were done in MHSP.
- Of the 18% of women patients who did not receive a Pap smear, 75% had a cervix and thus would have benefited from screening.

Informal Discussion:

- Gynecology teaching occurred in an inconsistent and haphazard manner in relation to a resident's clinical experience.
- A gynecology elective was available but was viewed as being poorly organized. It was only occasionally taken by residents, predominantly GIM residents.

■ Curricular time could be made available during the GIM residents' ambulatory block time.

Steps 1 and 2 confirmed the need for a primary care gynecology curriculum for internists, defined the targeted learners and location for the curriculum, and identified desired and needed content areas.

Step 3: Overall Goals of the Curriculum

An important area in thinking about this curriculum was identifying the interface between general internal medicine and obstetrics-gynecology; defining (a) the problems and procedures for which internists should be expected to have competency and (b) the guidelines for appropriate referrals. There was a paucity of literature on this interface, and the interface could be expected to vary depending on the community or health system in which the internist was practicing. The developers of this curriculum used the results of problem identification, needs assessments, expert opinion, and their own clinical experiences to identify the goals and objectives for this curriculum. They were tempered by resource constraints in terms of faculty and curricular time. For example, performance objectives were not included because the curriculum faculty did not have the resources to perform yearly audits. One important content area, breast examinations and breast cancer screening, was not included because it was covered elsewhere in the residency, and residents felt competent in this area.

Goals	■ To prepare residents to manage competently the primary care gynecologic needs of their patients, eliminating the need for unnecessary referrals to gynecologists.
	■ To give residents the knowledge base necessary to effectively triage patients with gynecologic emergencies.
	■ To have residents understand the evidence behind gynecologic screening tests and hormone replacement.
Objectives	*Cognitive Objectives:* At the completion of the gynecology curriculum, the following will be the result:
	■ 70% of participants will correctly identify appropriate diagnosis, management, and referral strategies for abnormal uterine bleeding, chronic pelvic pain, premenstrual syndrome, vaginitis/sexually transmitted diseases, domestic violence, and gynecologic emergencies.
	■ 70% of participants will identify and justify his or her use of a particular screening guideline for cervical cancer.
	■ 90% of participants will recite mechanism of action, two common side effects or inconveniences, and two counseling points for each broad category of contraceptive methods.
	■ 90% of participants will correctly identify candidates and outline management strategy for hormonal replacement therapy.
	■ 90% of participants will identify available resources for determining safe medications during pregnancy.
	■ 100% of participants will identify, based on the U.S. Preventive

Task Force Guidelines, appropriate candidates for pelvic examinations and Pap smears.

Affective Objectives: At completion of the gynecology curriculum, the following will be the result:

- 80% of participants will rate their competency in performing a pelvic and Pap examination as either good or excellent.
- 100% will believe that it is important for the primary care internist to be competent in providing gynecologic care for their female patients.
- 80% of participants will believe it is possible to deliver primary gynecologic care in a timely fashion, while also attending to the other health needs of their patients.

Psychomotor Objectives: By the end of the gynecology curriculum, the following will be the result:

- Each participant will have demonstrated the appropriate technique to perform a pelvic examination and to obtain a Pap smear and cervical cultures (*skill objective*).
- Each participant will demonstrate appropriate methods to determine whether a pregnant woman's cervical os is open (*skill objective*).
- Each participant will demonstrate the technique of wet prep slide preparation and potassium hydroxide slide preparation for the evaluation of common vaginal infections (*skill objective*).
- Each participant will have demonstrated at least two techniques of placing the patient at ease during the pelvic examination (*skill objective*).

Process Objectives:

- By the end of the gynecology curriculum, each GIM resident will have attended at least 90% of the didactic and clinical sessions.
- By the end of the second year of program implementation, 70% of residents attending at least 90% of didactic and clinical sessions will have rated the gynecology curriculum as good or excellent.

Step 4: Educational Strategies

Having specified learning objectives, the authors chose educational strategies that would facilitate the achievement of skill objectives through supervised clinical experience and that would facilitate the achievement of knowledge objectives through structured didactic sessions. Attitudinal objectives would be met through discussion and through improved comfort in managing gynecologic issues as the residents' experience and competency increased. Note that the content of the learning was chosen to match the learning objectives.

Content   Content areas include pelvic examinations; cervical cancer screening and the initial management of abnormal Pap smears;

overview of other pelvic malignancies; contraception; pregnancy-preconception counseling and medications; premenstrual syndrome; vaginitis and sexually transmitted diseases; domestic violence; abnormal uterine bleeding; chronic pelvic pain; menopause and hormone replacement therapy; gynecologic emergencies, including pelvic inflammatory disease and ectopic pregnancy.

Methods

Lectures/Discussions: 1- to 1½-hour lecture/discussion sessions on each topic area. Responsibilities for different content areas divided among faculty. Lectures videotaped for use when responsible faculty member not available and for use by residents as needed.

Syllabus Material: Concise, practical, clinically relevant handouts for each content area. Skills checklist for pelvic examination and obtaining Pap smear.

Clinical Experience:
- Supervised clinical experience in a gynecology setting three sessions per week for one month of each resident's training; emphasis on techniques of doing pelvic examinations and obtaining Pap smears.
- GIM clinical experience: (a) community-based practice experience structured to expect and support the efficient provision of primary gynecologic care by the internist; (b) support staff in MHSP primed to assist during pelvic examinations, although incorporation of pelvic examinations is expected to remain inefficient until completion of a new ambulatory building.

Step 5: Implementation

The authors met with the GIM Residency Program Director and determined that the ideal time for the curriculum would be during the residents' ambulatory block rotations. The block rotations included four half-days of community-based GIM practice, one half-day of MHSP, one half-day of visits to a home care panel of patients, three half-days of related subspecialty clinical experience, and one half-day of didactics. One quarter of PGY-2 and -3 residents were in an ambulatory block rotation on any given month. The didactic curriculum was, therefore, repeated for four consecutive months every two years. The gynecology clinical experience takes place in three sessions per week during most months of the year. It was felt that concurrent general internal medicine community-based practice experiences would permit residents to apply newly acquired gynecologic competencies in their general internal medicine practices.

Resources

Personnel: Faculty
- Curriculum development: Two internist clinician-educator faculty, one internist medical education fellow, one gynecologist faculty, and one gynecology fellow met for two to four hours per week for about nine months to develop and pilot parts of the curriculum.

- Gynecology clinical experience: Three clinic sessions per week are precepted by a gynecology faculty member.
- Lectures/discussions: 14 to 16 hours per month, plus preparation time, for four months every two years, divided among faculty members.

Personnel: Support staff: Gynecology and GIM secretaries spend one to four hours per month constructing schedules and copying syllabus materials. They also spend a few hours at the end of the year tallying evaluation results.

Facilities: Conference room for lecture/discussion and a clinic space for gynecologic examinations.

Equipment: A pelvic model; videotape equipment to tape lectures.

Funding: The Faculty Development Program, which includes workshops on curriculum development and curriculum mentors, was supported in part by a federal grant. Partial salary support from a federal GIM residency grant was provided to one internist and one gynecologist during the development period, and to one gynecologist during the first year of implementation. Currently, Gynecology and GIM have an arrangement whereby each provides faculty time to the other's residency program so that no funds are exchanged. The pelvic model was obtained with grant funds. The GIM division provides the videotaping equipment.

Support	*External Support:* The development and implementation of a primary care gynecology curriculum was supported in part by a federal grant obtained by the GIM Residency Program.
	Internal Support: GIM Division Co-Chiefs, GIM Residency Grant Project Director, and GIM Residency Director commissioned and strongly support the curriculum. Internist faculty remove an hour from their clinical schedule for each hour spent teaching in the gynecology curriculum. Residents had requested and strongly support the curriculum.
Administration	One internist serves as the Curriculum Coordinator. She coordinates the lecture/discussion series, the updating of syllabus material, the review of evaluation results, and communication among faculty regarding the curriculum. A GIM secretary assists in scheduling the lectures/discussions, copying syllabus material, and tallying evaluation results. A gynecology secretary coordinates the scheduling of gynecologic clinic sessions with the GIM secretary and gynecology faculty.
Barriers	*Faculty from Outside the Department/Division:* The devotion of faculty time from other departments/divisions was secured initially by direct payment and later by a mutually beneficial commitment

(see above). Without such arrangements, it was felt that the contribution of uncompensated faculty time would be subject to withdrawal in the face of other demands for faculty time.

Loss of an Externally Supported Family Planning Clinic: After a hiatus of one month, a suitable replacement was found for one of the principal sites of the residents' clinical training in gynecology.

Faculty Turnover: The development of a team of internists and gynecologists who have been involved in the development and implementation of the curriculum has permitted the curriculum to manage transient and permanent faculty turnover.

Introduction	The curriculum was developed as a *mentored project* in the Johns Hopkins Faculty Development Program for Clinician Educators (FDP) during 1993–1994. The curriculum was constructed after a careful needs assessment and the assurance of divisional and resident support. The full curriculum was *piloted* before full implementation *upon other team members.* Some lectures/discussions were piloted upon *colleagues* in the FDP. The Gynecology clinical experience was piloted on two *interested interns.* The curriculum was *fully implemented on all PGY-2 and -3 GIM residents* during 1994–1995.

Step 6: Evaluation

Because of limited resources, the evaluation has been kept simple. Data collection is integrated into the curriculum schedule. The major goals of the evaluation are to provide formative information that the residents can use to achieve curricular objectives and that the faculty can use to monitor the quality of and to improve the curriculum. Time and resources are not allocated to tally pretest data; pretest data are used solely for formative individual evaluation.

Users	Residents, curriculum faculty, GIM residency director, department chair/overall residency program director.
Uses	Formative information to help residents achieve learning objectives; formative information for the curriculum coordinator and faculty to guide improvement of curriculum; summative information for the GIM residency director on program effectiveness/worthiness of continued support; summative information to help the department chair/residency program directors assess individual performance.
Resources	Curriculum faculty and secretaries. No additional funding.
Evaluation questions	What percentage of residents scored ≥85% on the knowledge posttest? What percentage of residents were able to perform a

competent, supervised pelvic examination as determined by their supervisor? What are the strengths of the curriculum? What are its weaknesses? How can the curriculum be improved?

Evaluation Designs	$O_1 - - - X - - - O_2$: Knowledge test, pelvic examination competency checklist (formative individual)
	$X --- O$: Knowledge test (summative program) Pelvic examination competency checklist (summative individual and program) End of rotation Department of Medicine global evaluation form on each resident, completed by gynecology clinical attending (summative individual)

Evaluation Methods and Instruments

Gynecology Knowledge Test: A multiple choice knowledge test that covers the most important knowledge objectives of the curriculum. Residents self-administer and grade the test at the beginning of the lecture/discussion series. At the end of the curriculum, residents take the same test, grade it, and hand it in unsigned. The test serves as a formative evaluation tool for each resident (formative individual evaluation) by focusing the residents on the key content of the curriculum and providing them with the correct answers after taking the test. By tallying the results of the anonymous posttests for all residents, the test permits faculty to determine how effective their lectures/discussions were in achieving learner cognitive objectives (summative program evaluation).

Pelvic Examination Competency Checklist: Residents are given a lecture on the pelvic examination and receive a copy of the checklist. The attending gynecologist observes the resident performing the pelvic examination early in the rotation and administers the checklist to highlight areas of performance strengths and weaknesses (formative individual evaluation). The attending gynecologist observes the resident again at the end of the rotation and completes a checklist. The latter provides both feedback for the resident and information that the attending gynecologist uses in completing the Department of Medicine end-of-rotation global evaluation form (formative and summative individual evaluation). Results are pooled for summative program evaluation. Patients give informed consent for the exams.

Standard Department of Medicine Global Evaluation Form: Completed by a gynecology faculty member at the end of the clinical experience. It rates residents on several attribute scales (e.g., knowledge; independent learning; gathering of clinical information; quality of notes; presentation of clinical data; clinical reasoning ability and judgment; responsibility, initiative, and motivation; organization and efficiency; rapport with patients and family; patient education; relations with co-workers; humaneness of patient care; ability to take and respond to constructive criticism; integrity; required reading) and asks for written comments on strengths, weaknesses, and areas/suggestions for improvement.

End of Curriculum Evaluation Form: Elicits residents' ratings of the adequacy with which each content area has been covered, written comments on curriculum strengths, suggestions for improvements, and opinions about whether residents would recommend the curriculum to others ("no," or "yes" as a "satisfactory," "good," or "outstanding" experience).

Ethical Concerns	Patients are made aware of the learner evaluation process and are asked to consent prior to evaluation pelvic examinations. Residents perform pelvic examinations without supervision only after the attending gynecologist is convinced of their competence. End-of-curriculum evaluation forms are completed by residents anonymously to promote uninhibited ratings and comments and to protect residents against any retaliation for unflattering ratings or comments.
Data Collection	End-of-curriculum knowledge tests are administered and collected during the last lecture/discussion session. End-of-curriculum evaluation forms are collected at the end of each year in order to permit assessment of both the lecture/discussion series and the clinical component of training, which may be temporally disconnected (see above). Global evaluation forms are returned to the chair of the Department of Medicine by the attending gynecologist at the end of the clinical component of the rotation.
Data Analysis	Knowledge posttests and end-of-curriculum evaluation forms are tallied by the GIM residency secretary. Written comments are transcribed verbatim. Results are reviewed and discussed yearly by the curriculum faculty.
Reporting of Results	Tallied results of the posttest knowledge tests and end-of-curriculum evaluation forms, along with verbatim comments, are shared with the GIM residency director.

Curriculum Maintenance and Enhancement

The major anticipated challenge is to maintain a viable, enthusiastic team of faculty who periodically update and revise the curriculum to meet evolving needs.

Understanding the Curriculum and Managing Change	It is the job of the curriculum coordinator to maintain a good understanding of the curriculum through review of evaluation results, occasional observation of sessions other than her own, and discussion with curriculum faculty, residents, and the GIM residency director (who receives feedback from residents). The curriculum

coordinator makes minor changes herself, such as schedule changes, and coordinates faculty meetings to make substantive changes in the curriculum.

Sustaining the Curriculum Team/ Related Activities That Strengthen the Curriculum	*Networking/Scholarly Activity:* The curriculum team has *presented portions of the lecture/discussion curriculum at two national meetings* of the Society of General Internal Medicine (SGIM) and *at a regional continuing medical education course* for practicing primary care clinicians. The team won a junior faculty award for education at one of the SGIM meetings. Currently the curriculum coordinator is coediting a book and faculty members are contributing chapters to a multiauthored book on gynecology for the internist, which is scheduled to be published by the American College of Physicians.

Dissemination

Based on their problem identification and general needs assessment (Step 1), the curriculum developers anticipated a broad audience for their curriculum among primary care clinicians. The lecture/discussion component could be delivered to large audiences and seemed suitable for dissemination.

Target Audience	Practicing primary care practitioners and generalist practitioners in training.
Reasons for Dissemination	The major reasons were to help address the health care problem identified in Step 1, to motivate and invigorate the curricular team, and to help the curriculum developers to achieve recognition and academic advancement. A further benefit has been enrichment through interchange and collaboration with colleagues. For example, the request for a book, and an expanded group of collaborators, resulted from workshop/minicourse presentations at a national meeting (see above).
Content	The content for dissemination has been the curricular material itself. There is a need for practical, evidence-based, well-organized presentations of gynecology and women's health topics that are oriented to primary care clinicians. The curricular evaluation was designed for internal and predominantly formative purposes and was not thought to have the scientific rigor that would make it appropriate for dissemination. The literature search for Step 1 was limited; and although an original needs assessment of targeted residents was performed, it was not felt that it was sufficiently representative of residents or practicing internists to warrant dissemination.
Methods	*Workshops/Minicourses:* See above (Curriculum Maintenance and Enhancement).

Book: See above (Curriculum Maintenance and Enhancement).
Distribution of Curricular Materials on Request

Resources	Secretarial support and funds for travel have been provided by the GIM division and the faculty group practice.

AMBULATORY CLERKSHIP IN
GENERAL INTERNAL MEDICINE FOR MEDICAL STUDENTS

In 1995, the Dean of Academic Affairs charged the Department of Medicine at the Johns Hopkins University School of Medicine to develop an ambulatory experience for medical students in internal medicine. In response, the Department of Medicine Chair convened a task force of educational faculty from the Department of Medicine at Johns Hopkins Hospital and five of its affiliated local institutions to explore the feasibility of a clerkship, and, if feasible, to develop one. A task force of faculty in the department worked for nine months to design a three-week experience in ambulatory internal medicine, which was implemented in the spring of 1996. The faculty primarily responsible for the curriculum are Patricia Thomas, M.D.; Maura Maguire, M.D.; and Lucille King, M.D. Numerous others have contributed to its development and implementation.

Compared to the residency curriculum in primary care gynecology, this curriculum was broader and less differentiated in its goals and objectives. The curriculum planners were allotted three weeks for the clerkship. The curriculum would require a decentralized format and nearly as many faculty preceptors as students taking the clerkship. This clerkship addresses some of the challenges of curriculum development for clinical training (1, 2) in that the type of patients, problems, and preceptors were destined to differ for each student, resulting in a qualitatively different clinical experience for each student. Content-specific knowledge and skill and attitudinal learning objectives were less appropriate here than (a) helping students to develop an approach to patients and problems in outpatient settings and (b) generating an enthusiasm for internal medicine as practiced in ambulatory settings.

Step 1: Problem Identification and General Needs Assessment

Because the charge to the task force was to develop an ambulatory clerkship for medical students, the general needs assessment focused upon current and ideal approaches to medical student training. An important goal of the task force was to identify well-constructed current work in the area, in order to avoid "reinventing the wheel." The problem identification was used to put the general needs assessment into perspective.

In addition to a review of the medical literature, the curriculum developers were helped by accessing other sources of available information. Especially helpful was the *Core Medicine Clerkship Curriculum Guide,* developed jointly by the Society of General Internal Medicine (SGIM) and the Clerkship Directors of Internal Medicine (CDIM) (3). The authors of this guide used a consensus of national faculty to identify and prioritize competencies for students in the third-year internal medicine clerkship. The authors also addressed educational strategies, evaluation, and faculty development. While the new clerkship would address only the ambulatory component, the model curriculum was a helpful beginning. Other useful resources included materials from the American College of Physicians (4, 5) and the American Society of Internal Medicine (ASIM) (6).

Problem Identification	In 1995 the United States faced a shortage of generalist physicians. Internists provide the largest proportion of primary adult care in the United States, yet internal medicine training programs have produced a disproportionate number of specialists compared to generalists.

Most medical students choose their career path during the third and fourth years of training, based upon their experiences in their core clinical clerkships. Over the previous decade, there had been a steady fall in the number of students opting for careers in internal medicine. Studies showed that a majority of students who were seriously considering a career in internal medicine changed their minds after their internal medicine core clerkship. Family practice was rising in popularity among students as a career choice.

There was a mismatch between internal medicine residency training and societal needs. Economic realities and managed care have increased demands for and capabilities of caring for patients outside acute hospitals, demands for customer service and quality in ambulatory settings, demands for the integration of preventive care, and demands for an evidence-based, cost-effective, coordinated approach to care whatever the setting. Internists, and physicians in general, have not been well trained in the practice of patient-centered, cost-effective, evidence-based, preventive care, particularly in ambulatory settings.

Many patients experience fragmented, patient-unfriendly, and cost-ineffective care, lack of access to high-quality generalist care, and a lack of preventive care.

Society experiences the health and economic consequences of the above, and lacks the generalist physician resources to correct the problem.

Current Approach	*Society:* Market forces are driving residents and student to pursue generalist careers rather than subspecialty careers. There are increasing demands for physicians who practice cost-effective medicine, interact well with patients, and work well with physician and nonphysician colleagues in complex medical organizations.

Physicians: Many students and residents receive the bulk of their training in inpatient settings, with little exposure to intellectually and professionally satisfying models of general internal medicine practice and with little training in the skills necessary to successfully practice in today's complex, increasingly managed care health delivery system.

Medical Educators: Traditionally, internal medicine clerkships have been inpatient based. Students are taught primarily by house staff, who are often overworked and discouraged and whose clinical experience is predominantly inpatient based. Inpatient experiences, which are not representative of internal medicine practice in general, have become characterized by increased patient volumes per resident, a skewed spectrum of illnesses, increased severity of illness, shortened length of stays, preplanned admissions with management approaches already decided, and an emphasis on interventional and intensive care. Students who change their minds about a career in internal medicine cite as reasons demoralized house staff and attendings, a discouraging spectrum of patients and illnesses, heavy workload, and little opportunity to develop relationships with patients.

Ideal Approach	A third-year internal medicine clerkship should train students in settings that:

- Expose students to a mix of patients, patient problems, and physician skills that are representative of internal medicine practice
- Emphasize clinical decision making by using an intellectual rigor that is traditional to internal medicine
- Emphasize the development of communication skills and longitudinal relationships with patients

The clerkship should include, in addition to an inpatient experience, an ambulatory experience in community-based practices, with faculty mentors/preceptors who are clinically astute and enthusiastic about their profession.

Step 2: Needs Assessment of Targeted Learners

The curriculum developers began by identifying students' other learning experiences that might relate to an ambulatory internal medicine clerkship. It was realized that as students progressed through their clinical years they would arrive at this clerkship with different previous clinical experiences, levels of maturation, and learning needs. It was decided, therefore, to integrate a needs assessment of individual learners into the educational and evaluation strategies of the clerkship itself by the use of a self-assessment form, individualized learning contracts, a clinical experience log, and an ongoing process of observation by and discussion with a clinical preceptor. Part of the faculty development for the clerkship includes introducing clinical preceptors to the concept of the learning contract and encouraging them to use it to direct the clinical experiences of their students.

Targeted Learners	Third- and fourth-year medical students (clinical years).
Needs Assessment	*Background Information Known to Curriculum Developers:* During their second year, *all students* are trained in clinical skills (history and physical examination skills) and complete a practicum in evidence-based medicine and literature search skills.

Students will vary with respect to previous clinical clerkship experience. *Some students* will have completed their inpatient internal medicine clerkship. Some will have had ambulatory experiences in pediatrics, obstetrics-gynecology, and other clerkships. A few will be clinically inexperienced.

Self-Assessment Clinical Skills Inventory, Log of Clinical Experience, and Faculty Observation: These educational and formative evaluation strategies encourage the identification of individual needs.

Individualized Learning Contracts: These contracts are completed by each student at the beginning of the clerkship, after completion of the self-assessment clinical skills inventory, and in collaboration with their preceptor. The contract accommodates differences among students in past experience, learning needs, career paths and goals. For instance, a student interested in orthopedics might set a goal of improving his musculoskeletal examination and learning office injection techniques. The following is a sample of learning plan objectives listed by students in the first rotation of the clerkship:

- Learning screening and prevention strategies
- Listening to heart sounds and making relevant diagnoses
- Learning long-term management of diabetes and complications
- Learning to take a focused history and physical
- Gaining more experience with eyes, ears, nose, and throat examinations
- Learning differences between ambulatory and inpatient settings
- Understanding the managed care setting, including cost and time issues
- Interacting with patients, including assessing hidden agenda, abuse issues, etc.
- Improving skills, especially pelvic and cardiac examinations
- Improving skills in reading electrocardiograms
- Learning how to manage my time with patients.

Step 3: Overall Goals of the Curriculum

The SGIM/CDIM model curriculum was available as a reference. The task force process for defining goals included a brainstorming session during which learner goals were placed on flip charts, prioritized, and subsequently grouped into four general categories. Program goals and specific measurable objectives were developed to be congruent with the learner goals, a consensus goal that students view the role of the general internist positively, and the goal of maintaining a successful curriculum.

Goals   *Goals for Learners:* During the clerkship, each student will:
- Develop core generalist competencies:
  Care of the healthy patient, preventive medicine

Care of the patient with acute illnesses
Longitudinal care of the patient with chronic illnesses
Care through a complete illness
- Learn to think like an internist, with emphasis on:
   Diagnostic decision making
   Evidence-based, cost-effective medicine
   Self-directed learning
- Develop the skills of an internist:
   Communication with patients
   Communication with colleagues, ability to work in teams
   Comprehensive approach to patient care
   Skills useful in office practice, including urinalysis, pelvic ex-
      amination, arthrocentesis
- Develop a mentorship relationship with an internist role model:
   Ethical care of patients
   Lifelong learning
   Balance of professional responsibilities

Program Goals
- Students taking the ambulatory clerkship in medicine will achieve the generalist competencies noted above.
- Students will consider the ambulatory clerkship to be a positive learning experience and, in particular, will value the educational methods employed:
   Faculty preceptors and clinical experience
   Hospital-based conferences and skill-building exercises
   Learning portfolio
- Students will establish mentoring relationships with faculty.
- Students will appreciate the role of the general internist and will perceive internal medicine as an attractive career choice.
- Faculty will perceive their teaching and participation as a favorable and valued experience.

Objectives	*Cognitive Objectives:* By the end of the three-week clerkship, each student will have done the following: - Demonstrated an understanding of the evidence-based approach to clinical decision making by completing an evidence-based written report on a question of his/her choosing - Demonstrated understanding of an evidence-based, cost-effective approach to managing 10 common problems of ambulatory patients by successfully completing the self-test at the end of each section of the workbook - Considered the costs of common outpatient prescriptions and diagnostics in the care of patients by having noted these costs in the written case reports - Demonstrated the ability to direct aspects of one's own learning by the development and at least partial accomplishment of a learning contract

Psychomotor and Affective Objectives: By the end of the three-week clerkship, each student will have demonstrated the following:

- The ability to take a focused history and perform a focused physical examination for three common outpatient problems during a standardized patient examination
- The ability to effectively counsel a patient in a health-related behavior change
- A professional and humanistic approach to the care of patients as observed by his or her office preceptor in the clinical setting

By the end of the three-week clerkship:

- The percentage of students considering internal medicine as a career choice will be maintained or increased, compared to the percentage at the beginning of the clerkship.

Process Objectives: By the end of the three-week clerkship,

- ≥ 70% of students will have had a relationship with a preceptor that addressed professional-personal issues such as ethical considerations in patient care, continued learning, and the balance of professional and personal responsibilities.
- Students and clinical preceptors, on average, will rate each component of the clerkship ≥ 3 on a 4-point scale and will recommend participation in the clerkship to colleagues as a "good" or "outstanding" experience (as opposed to a "satisfactory" or "not recommended" experience).

Step 4: Educational Strategies

Educational strategies were chosen that were congruent with the goals for learners that are listed above.

Content

Content depends in large part on the students' clinical experience at their practice sites. For most sites, it should reflect the epidemiology of general internal medicine practice and should include preventive care, the care of patients with acute illnesses, and the care of patients with chronic conditions (see goals). The patient logs maintained by the students permit retrospective analysis of an individual student's experience, as well as the range of experience provided by a practice site. In addition, 10 content areas are included in the students' workbook of ambulatory problems: health promotion and counseling; screening and prevention; cough; dysuria; low back pain; anemia; hypertension; diabetes mellitus; smoking cessation; depression. Content areas were chosen based on the following criteria: the degree to which the areas were representative of the epidemiology of ambulatory practice, the degree to which the areas would embody the learning goals for the clerkship, and the identification of a faculty member who was willing to prepare a workbook section on that topic.

Methods

Patient-Based Learning: Students are assigned to community-based internal medicine practices, with volunteer part-time faculty preceptors. Students are expected to attend at least five half-day sessions per week in their community practices. A sixth clinical session may be either at the community practice or in a subspecialty clinic. It is expected that students will see 30 to 60 patient encounters over the three-week experience. Preceptors are advised that they should expose students to a spectrum of outpatient problems, including examination and counseling of healthy patients, care of patients with acute problems, and patients with chronic conditions. (Note the relationship of this method to the first of the goals for learners.)

Case Write-Ups: Students are asked to submit three case write-ups of patients seen during the clerkship. Students are told to address the psychosocial aspects of illness and include costs of all medications and diagnostic tests. Lastly, they are instructed to list the learning points they experienced in each case.

Small-Group Learning: Twice a week, students assemble in small groups of six to eight, with faculty facilitators, for interactive teaching sessions. Three of these sessions are devoted to communication and medical interview skills, and three to case-based discussions emphasizing clinical decision making and evidence-based medicine in outpatient settings. (It was felt that skill building in a sensitive area, such as communication skills, would be best accomplished in the safe environment of a properly facilitated small group, which works together over time as a learning team.)

Workbook of Ambulatory Problems: Using the prioritized competencies from the SGIM/CDIM core model curriculum, 10 outpatient topics were chosen by the curriculum developers for emphasis during this clerkship (see above). For each topic, an abbreviated introduction was written, an evidence-based practice guideline was supplied where appropriate, and a self-test was included. Students are told that they are expected to complete all 10 modules by the end of the clerkship.

The Learning Contract: At the orientation to the clerkship, students are asked to complete an inventory of clinical skills and subsequently to list three personal learning objectives for the clerkship with strategies for accomplishing them. Each student is instructed to show this learning plan to his or her preceptor, who will add or modify objectives; and the student and preceptor sign the contract on the first day of the clerkship. By identifying goals early, it is hoped that individual specific learning needs will be met.

Evidence-Based Report: Students are asked to choose one clinical question that arose during the clerkship and search the literature for an appropriate reference, critically appraise the article, and apply it to the case in question. A written report is required at the end of the clerkship. (The learning contract and the evidence-based report are educational strategies chosen to reinforce one goal of the clerkship: self-directed and lifelong learning.)

Independent Learning: Students are scheduled one-half day per week to work on their evidence-based reports, pursue aspects of their learning contracts, and maintain and review a *learning portfolio,* which contains the learning contract, the patient log, case write-ups, and an evidence-based report.

Standardized Patients: Although originally designed as a summative evaluation instrument, the standardized patient interactions provide an end-of-clerkship opportunity for the application of what has been learned and for feedback on skills (see below).

Step 5: Implementation

The task force submitted a budget and written plan for the clerkship to the dean and department chair. Once the clerkship was approved, the task force structured a time line of events for the first year, which included the following: development of an organizational structure for the clerkship and its evaluation; recruitment of faculty; orientation of students, faculty preceptors, and clinic sites to the curriculum and its process; faculty development; recruitment and training of simulated patients; and publishing of the workbook and assorted materials for preceptors and students.

Resources

Personnel:
Faculty

- Curriculum development: An average of eight faculty met for one hour monthly for nine months, two codirectors spent an extra 20 hours apiece preparing for the meetings and synthesizing the work of the group.
- Clerkship director and regional directors: One clerkship director, 0.1 FTE; three regional directors, 0.1 FTE.
- Clinical preceptors: 25 to 30 preceptors per quarter; five half-day sessions per week. Most are part-time faculty whose principal career focus is clinical practice.
- Small-group facilitators and seminar leaders: Six facilitators per site, each doing one 2-hour session per clerkship.
- Workbook faculty: Individual faculty undertook responsibility for writing modules for the workbook of ambulatory problems. Three cases were developed for standardized patients by authors of the corresponding modules in the workbook.
- Faculty orientation, communication, and development: One dinner meeting each year. Goals, objectives, educational and evaluation strategies are reviewed. Previous experiences are discussed, and faculty issues are addressed. Fortunately, a large percentage of the faculty, including preceptors, had already participated in a 10-month half-day-per-week, faculty development program that included training in personal time management,

feedback, small-group teaching, one-on-one precepting, interviewing, lecturing, and management skills.

Standardized Patients: Six standardized patients for eight hours per day, two days per clerkship, five clerkships per year. Several hours training for each standardized patient initially, with follow-up as needed. A few hours per clerkship for administrative coordination and scheduling of patients. All functions are coordinated through a medical school education center.

Support Staff: 0.2 FTE secretary for clerkship director; three 0.1 FTE regional secretaries.

Facilities and Equipment: Conference rooms for six to seven people two half-days per week for small-group learning at each regional site; clinical sites must provide a separate examining room for each student; audio and visual equipment for small-group communication skills learning and for standardized patient interactions.

Funding: Partial funding support from the dean's office to pay for the time of the clerkship director and her secretary, for the standardized patient evaluations, and for production of the course syllabus.

Support	*External Support:* SGIM/CDIM guidelines provided support for the focus, content, and methods of the curriculum.

Internal Support
- Dean: A curricular plan was written and submitted to the dean with a budget. The dean then carved out curricular time for the clerkship and designated it a required clinical clerkship. The School of Medicine Clinical Education Center provides the standardized patient evaluations.
- Department chair: The chair assigned faculty time and resources to the development of the curriculum, and supported faculty status and other incentives for preceptors.
- Regional chairs: The time of the regional directors, faculty members, and secretaries was contributed by the Chiefs of Medicine at affiliated hospital sites.
- Community practices: Donate space and preceptor time. The medical directors of the major contributing practice groups were involved in the clerkship development process or had professional relationships with those who were involved.

Administration	*Administrative Structure:* A clerkship director is responsible for coordinating the overall clerkship. The clerkship is split into three regional sites, with assigned regional directors. The regional directors oversee the assignment of students to local preceptors, the scheduling and implementation of the small-group sessions at each regional site, and the evaluation of the students' learning portfolios.

Communication and Operations: Approximately two weeks before the start of the clerkship, the clerkship director is notified by the medical school registrar of the students who are assigned to clerkship. The clerkship director reviews students' addresses and assigns the students to one of three regional sites based on zip codes. Regional directors then assign the students to community preceptors, and the directors make up and distribute the schedule of small-group meetings at each regional site. Students meet with the clerkship director on the first day of the clerkship for orientation and meet with regional directors on the final day for feedback and evaluation. The clerkship director distributes the syllabi/workbooks at orientation, arranges the standardized patient examinations through the education center for the last week of the clerkship, coordinates evaluation activities, and produces and distributes evaluation reports. The clerkship and regional secretaries assist the clerkship and regional directors in these activities and ensure the distribution and collection of all evaluation instruments.

Barriers

Recruitment of Faculty: It was quickly identified that a limiting factor would be the availability of preceptors willing to take students into their practices and to devote additional time to teaching. Lists of existing and potential part-time faculty were generated. Incentives were proposed and approved: faculty appointment, free registration at department-sponsored continuing education courses, a textbook of medicine, and a recognition plaque.

Scheduling: The medical school has linked this three-week ambulatory clerkship to a six-week obstetrics-gynecology clerkship in order to complete a nine-week scheduling block. Student decisions regarding the scheduling of obstetrics-gynecology, therefore, affect the scheduling of the ambulatory internal medicine clerkship, which is not linked to the nine-week inpatient internal medicine clerkship. If the ambulatory clerkship is taken during the fourth year of medical school, its influence on career choice will be limited.

Evaluation: The medical school registrar requires that a uniform School of Medicine student evaluation form be completed by preceptors at the end of the clerkship, one that is tied only loosely to the goals and objectives of the clerkship. It was felt to be unwise to ask preceptors to complete two separate evaluation forms on the students. Therefore, preceptors do not consistently provide input on learner performance related to some specific curricular objectives (e.g., "Think like an internist").

Introduction

The curriculum was fully implemented in April 1996, as a required clerkship, and was refined, based upon formative evaluation results, over the first few cycles. The standardized patient examination was piloted in the first rotation and became a part of the final grading system by the second rotation.

Step 6: Evaluation

Evaluation methods were chosen that were congruent with curriculum objectives and educational strategies. The use of learning contracts, self-assessments, and workbook self-tests permit students to see if learning objectives have been met. Patient logs permit students to see the case mix and breadth of outpatient medicine and permit the regional directors to assess the adequacy of the clinical experience that is provided at each site. The use of case write-ups and an evidence-based report permit demonstration of an evidence-based, cost-effective approach to clinical decision making. The cases for the standardized patient examination are selected from the workbook on ambulatory problems; in addition to knowledge base, the cases test the skill of performing a focused history and physical examination and the application of preventive strategies. The preceptor evaluation, which includes the subjective components of professionalism and humanism, counts for 50% of the student grade. Clerkship and preceptor evaluation forms provide information on the accomplishment of process objectives and provide feedback that can be used for continued improvement of the clerkship. Questions that are integrated into the above evaluation instruments assess the influence of the clerkship on student attitudes regarding internal medicine as a career.

Users and Uses	*Students:* Formative information to provide students with feedback regarding the achievement of learning objectives and direction for further learning; summative information for students to include in their learning portfolios.
	Clinical Preceptors and Site Medical Directors: Formative information to provide feedback on preceptor and site performance and suggestions for improvement; summative information for faculty to include in their teaching portfolios.
	Curriculum Faculty: Formative information to provide feedback and suggestions for improvement in small-group learning sessions; summative information for teaching portfolios.
	Curriculum Coordinators and Regional Directors: Formative information on various curricular components to help direct improvements; summative information on individual learners to permit the assignment of grades; summative information on individual faculty, sites, and curricular components to guide decisions regarding the continued inclusion or the need for further development of those faculty, sites, and components; summative information on overall program effectiveness to justify continued support from dean and department chair; summative information for teaching portfolios.
	Department Chair and Dean of Academic Affairs: Summative information on curricular effectiveness to justify continued support or to identify the need for further development/intervention.
Resources	Standardized patients, curriculum faculty, and secretaries (see Step 5). Office supplies and equipment. No external funding.

Evaluation Questions	▪ What are the strengths and weaknesses of the curriculum? How can the curriculum be improved?

Evaluation Questions

▪ What are the strengths and weaknesses of the curriculum? How can the curriculum be improved?
▪ Will students and preceptors find the ambulatory clerkship in internal medicine enjoyable and productive?
▪ Will the percentage of students considering internal medicine as a career be maintained or increased?
▪ What grade should be assigned to each student?
▪ What percentage of students completing the ambulatory clerkship in medicine will score more than 80% on a standardized patient (SP) checklist of history and physical examination items for a case of essential hypertension?
▪ What percentage of students completing the ambulatory clerkship in medicine will demonstrate competency in counseling skills as demonstrated by performance in a standardized patient case of smoking cessation?
▪ What percentage of students will correctly diagnose clinical depression in a standardized patient who presents with insomnia?
▪ What percentage of students will complete a learning portfolio and the evidence-based medicine report to demonstrate the skills of self-directed learning, literature searching, and critical appraisal of literature?

Evaluation Designs and Methods

$O_1 - - - X_1 - - - O_2 - - - \ldots - - - X_{n-1} - - - O_n$:
Ongoing faculty *observation* and *feedback* throughout the clerkship, which includes beginning-of-clerkship and middle-of-clerkship *meetings* to discuss learning contracts and to review learning portfolios (formative individual evaluation).

$O_1 - - - X - - - O_2$:
Self-assessment instrument (clinical skill inventory) that is completed by each student (formative individual evaluation).
Career interest question (summative program evaluation).

$X - - - O$:
Under this heading are the following:
▪ *A student evaluation form completed by clinical preceptors* (50% of grade) (summative individual evaluation)
▪ *A review-of-learning portfolio completed by the region director* (learning plan; patient log; case write-ups, evidence-based report, workbook self-tests, self-assessments) (25% of grade) (summative individual and program evaluation)
▪ *Standardized patient examinations* (simulated patients complete a checklist; students review checklists and videotapes of their cases with the regional director) (25% of grade) (formative and summative individual and program evaluation)
▪ *Clerkship evaluation forms completed by students on the last day of the clerkship and by the preceptors annually* (formative and summative program evaluation)

- *Clinical preceptor and site evaluation forms completed by students on the last day of the clerkship* (formative and summative program evaluation)
- *Informal feedback elicited from students during end of clerkship meeting with regional directors* (formative program evaluation)

Ethical Concerns	*Confidentiality and Access:* Clerkship evaluation forms are completed anonymously by students and preceptors. Feedback to individual preceptors, based on preceptor and site evaluation forms, is provided after several forms have been completed in order to protect the confidentiality of the student respondents. Results of standardized patient examinations and learning portfolios are reviewed with the students at the end of the rotation and are returned to the students after grading sheets have been completed by the regional directors.
	Resource Allocation: Almost all of the curriculum's limited resources are used for teaching support, necessary program administration, and evaluation activities that are required (e.g., the assignment of grades), that have educational value for the students, or that provide feedback that fosters improvement of the curriculum. Resources have not been devoted to a sophisticated data analysis or evaluation design or to an attempt to assess outcomes.
Data Collection	Learning portfolios (learning plans, patient logs, case write-ups, evidence-based reports, workbook self-tests, self-assessments) are reviewed with students in end-of-clerkship meetings with the regional directors and are graded after the meeting. Regional secretaries distribute the preceptor, student, and clerkship evaluation forms. The student-completed preceptor and clerkship evaluation forms are returned to the regional secretaries at the time of the students' end-of-clerkship meetings with the regional directors. Clinical preceptors mail in their student and clerkship evaluation forms to the clerkship secretary. The clerkship secretary follows up if evaluation forms are not received within a short period after completion of the clerkship.
Data Analysis	Learning portfolios are reviewed and graded by the regional directors, using a portfolio evaluation sheet, and then are returned to the students. Performance checklists from the simulated patient examinations are reviewed and graded by the regional directors. Portfolio evaluation sheets, performance checklists from the simulated patient examinations, student and preceptor evaluation forms, and clerkship evaluation forms are tallied by the clerkship director. Written comments from the clerkship evaluation forms are transcribed verbatim. Results are analyzed by using descriptive statistics.

Reporting of Results	Grades are sent to the dean's office. Tallied evaluation results are distributed after each clerkship to the clerkship director, the regional directors, small-group facilitators, the department chair, and the dean. Tallied preceptor evaluation forms are reviewed with preceptors annually.

Curriculum Maintenance and Enhancement

Management of change is built into the administrative, operational, and evaluation structure of the clerkship. A major challenge is to maintain a large number of talented preceptors, who contribute time and practice resources for the clerkship.

Understanding the Curriculum and Managing Change	The clerkship director and regional directors manage minor changes in an ongoing fashion. They meet quarterly to review student performance and feedback and to decide on substantive changes in the curriculum. These meetings have resulted in the following changes: several sections of the workbook have been revised; some preceptors have been eliminated from the clerkship; and the simulated patient examination has been used increasingly for formative evaluation (learning) purposes. In the second year, fourth-year students are being included in the clerkship. It is anticipated that this change will alter the dynamics of the small-group learning sessions.
Sustaining the Curriculum Team/ Related Activities That Strengthen the Curriculum	Student evaluations are shared with teaching faculty and preceptors. There are incentives to encourage continued participation by the preceptors: faculty appointment, free registration at department-sponsored continuing education courses, a textbook of medicine, and a recognition plaque. There is an annual dinner retreat to discuss clerkship-related issues and to share preceptor experience, elicit feedback, and maintain enthusiasm for teaching. Targeted faculty development activities may be included in the retreats. Because it is difficult to get all faculty members together at one time in one place, other means of ongoing communication are being explored. For example, the clerkship director is working with the medical school informatics office to develop a web-based home page for the clerkship.

Dissemination

While this curriculum has not yet progressed to a stage of dissemination, it is important to note that it has benefited by the curricular work done by others, as noted in Step 1 of this example. It is also interesting to note that an important resource, the SGIM/CDIM curriculum guide, benefited from the active collaboration of educators from many institutions, and addresses Steps 1, 3, 4, 5, and 6 of the curriculum development process.

RESIDENCY TRAINING IN INTERVIEWING SKILLS AND THE PSYCHOSOCIAL DOMAIN OF MEDICAL PRACTICE

This curriculum, called the "Med-Psych Rotation," was implemented in 1979 at the Johns Hopkins Bayview Medical Center. Faculty primarily responsible for the development of this curriculum have included L. Randol Barker, M.D., Sc.M.; Karan A. Cole, Sc.D.; Archie S. Golden, M.D.; Marsha Grayson, M.A.; and David E. Kern, M.D., M.P.H. Several other faculty have contributed to developing the consultation liaison psychiatry, smoking cessation, and substance abuse components of the curriculum.* Not only has this curriculum progressed through all six stages of curriculum development, but it has also addressed issues related to curriculum maintenance, enhancement, and dissemination.

The curriculum was initially designed for pediatric and internal medicine residents. It included a seminar series, interviews of simulated patients, cointerviews of selected patients with a psychiatrist, and video reviews of ambulatory primary care patient visits. Two of the original faculty, a pediatrician and behavioral scientist, had developed a similar program for physician assistant students, so that much of the groundwork for the curriculum had already been developed. Progress on all steps proceeded simultaneously.

The program evolved during the first few years, based upon institutional changes such as the development of a consultation-liaison psychiatry service and the discontinuation of the pediatric residency program, and based upon evaluation results and feedback from residents. Early changes included the abandonment of lectures, an increase in the number of experimental learning exercises, establishment of a mutually beneficial role for residents and faculty in a new consultation-liaison psychiatry service, an increased emphasis on the recognition and management of psychosocial problems commonly seen in primary care practice, and an increased emphasis on the organization and efficiency of office visits. By 1983, the basic structure described below had been established.

Step 1: Problem Identification and General Needs Assessment

Literature searches were the major strategy for accomplishing this step. An in-depth literature review was conducted as part of a descriptive article on the rotation that was published in 1989 (7). One faculty member previously had conducted job and task analyses of primary care practice (8). Discussion among informed faculty members and interaction with colleagues from other institutions also contributed to the conceptualization of the ideal approach.

Problem Identification	<ul><li>Interviewing skills are critical to the establishment of an effective doctor-patient relationship, diagnosis, and patient management.</li><li>Psychosocial problems are common in medical practice.</li><li>Most of these psychosocial problems are not managed by mental health providers.</li><li>Psychosocial factors affect the management and outcomes of biomedical problems.</li></ul>

*Walter Baile, M.D.; Michael Fingerhood, M.D.; Carol Haines, M.D.; Lori Kreger, M.D.; Marsden Maguire, M.D.; Michael Mininsohn, M.D.; Theodore Parran, M.D.; Cynthia Rand, Ph.D.; Robert Roca, M.D.; and Penny Williamson, Sc.D.

- Psychosocial and biomedical aspects of health frequently cannot be separated.
- Physicians are frequently "hypocompetent" in interviewing skills and in the management of psychosocial components of care, with the consequences of poor patient satisfaction, malpractice suits, and suboptimal health outcomes.

Current Approach (1970s–1980s)

Society: There has been pressure from patient advocacy groups and from malpractice insurance carriers, and promotion by government agencies, medical professional organizations, and pharmaceutical companies (interest in patient compliance) to improve the training of physicians in these areas; and there has been pressure on physicians from managed care organizations and other insurers to improve physicians' communication skills, to improve patients' satisfaction, and simultaneously to become more efficient.

Patients: An increasingly educated and assertive patient population is more likely to demand information, to demand service, and to complain when their needs are not met. Patients are more likely to prefer a collaborative rather than an authoritative doctor–patient relationship.

Healthcare Providers: Physicians usually have been authoritative and physician-centered rather than patient centered in doctor–patient interactions, frequently have interrupted patients and ignored their concerns, frequently have accepted ill-defined complaints without clarification, frequently have not met patient educational or behavioral change needs. Physicians frequently have failed to recognize, have misdiagnosed, or have mismanaged the psychosocial problems of their patients.

Medical Educators: Effective techniques for teaching interviewing skills have been identified: real-time observation or video or audio reviews of trainee performance with real patients, simulated patients or role-plays, combined with feedback and discussion based on trainees' performance. Most medical schools, most family practice, and almost all federally funded primary care residency programs include training in interviewing skills and psychosocial medicine. Formal training is provided for a minority of pediatric residents. Traditional track internal medicine residents receive little training. Most training programs use at least one experiential educational method, but few use two or more. Simulated patients and role-plays are underutilized. Most medical school training is concentrated in the preclinical years. Interviewing skills training has emphasized data gathering and rapport building; organization, efficiency, patient education, behavioral counseling, office psychotherapy, and the ability to diagnose and manage the psychosocial problems that are common in medical practice are seldom addressed. Training is usually provided by behavioral scientists/psychiatrists and not by faculty who are in the same specialty as the trainees. Despite a shortage of adequately trained faculty, little attention has been paid in the literature to faculty development in this area. Funding and departmental support for training are often inadequate.

Ideal Approach

Physicians: Should be proficient in using communication skills to gather important information from patients, to build therapeutic relationships with patients, and to effectively educate and counsel patients. They should be proficient in recognizing, diagnosing, and managing psychosocial problems common in medical practice. They should be proficient in integrating the biomedical and psychosocial components of medical care.

Medical Educators should:
- Train all medical students and residents in the above proficiencies.
- Use effective educational methodologies, including two or more experiential learning methods.
- Cover content relevant to the training level and specialty.
- Include role model faculty in the same specialty that the trainees are in.
- Train faculty to teach effectively in this domain.
- Provide sufficient resources to accomplish the above.

Step 2: Needs Assessment of Targeted Learners

Based upon literature review, faculty experience with previous residents, and faculty knowledge of the existing residency program, the curriculum developers knew that (a) the residents' previous training as medical students in this area would be nonexistent to spotty, (b) most residents' mastery of the content area of the curriculum would be low, (c) learning needs would vary considerably among residents, and (d) residents received no formal training in this area in the existing residency. A formal precurriculum needs assessment of targeted learners was, therefore, thought to be unnecessary. It was decided, however, to integrate a needs assessment of targeted learners into the actual curriculum in order to address differences in the needs of individual learners.

Targeted Learners

PGY-1 (post-graduate year 1) residents. The first year of residency was chosen because it is a time when practice habits are being formed, when residents are likely to be looking for direction, and when residents have not yet developed defenses that interfere with learning.

Needs Assessment

Before implementation of the Med-Psych rotation, there was virtually no training in this domain in the residency program. Based upon information from the literature and *orientation meetings* with the residents on the rotation, training prior to residency was variable but usually minimal. Residents varied considerably in life experiences and baseline communication skills. At the beginning of each rotation, residents complete a *self-assessment instrument,* rating their perceived knowledge, their attitudes regarding importance, and their proficiencies in the content areas of the curriculum, and they identify their individual learning goals. Individual needs are also ascertained during experiential learning sessions by resident self-assessment and *faculty observation.*

Step 3: Goals and Objectives

The goals and objectives have evolved somewhat over the years. They derive directly from the general needs assessment described above. Individual objectives are defined in greater detail in syllabus material related to each content area and learning exercise.

Goals	The major goal of this curriculum is to help residents become humane and effective physicians by assisting them in developing their interviewing skills and their ability to recognize and manage patients' psychosocial problems. The curriculum concentrates on the types of patients and problems commonly seen in medical practice, so that what is learned can be applied, reinforced, and further developed as the residents mature. Related goals are to help residents become accurate assessors of their own feelings and behaviors with respect to patients and directors of their own learning in this area.
Objectives	*Cognitive Objectives:* By the end of the rotation, residents will have a clinically useful knowledge base in each of the following areas:

- Medical interview
- Psychosocial evaluation
- Psychotherapy/counseling
- Patient compliance with therapeutic regimens
- Smoking cessation management
- Alcoholism and coalcoholism
- Adjustment disorders
- Anxiety
- Depression and mood disorders
- Somatization and somatoform disorders
- Personality types and disorders
- Organic mental syndromes (dementia, delirium, determination of mental competence)
- Psychosis and psychiatric emergencies (e.g., assessment of suicide risk)

Affective Objectives: By the end of the rotation, residents will believe the following:

- An integrated biopsychosocial model of illness is more accurate than a dualistic, reductionist model that tries to separate the biomedical from the psychosocial.
- It is a physician's role to attend to the emotional and behavioral as well as the biomedical aspects of a patient's illness and health care.
- The cognitive and psychomotor skill objectives of the rotation are relevant and important.
- A collaborative, patient-centered approach to doctor–patient interactions is generally superior to an autocratic, physician-centered approach, and most interactions require a balance between the two.
- They are capable of providing patient-centered, biopsychosocial care to their patients; their skills in this domain have increased; and a patient-centered biopsychosocial approach to patient care is personally and professionally satisfying.

Psychomotor Objectives: By the end of the rotation, residents will have increased their proficiency in the following areas:
Interviewing skills:
- Using effective data-gathering methods: determining patient's agenda and concerns; using a balance of open-ended and focused questions; avoiding leading questions; using listening, responding, and observing skills
- Using affective/relationship building skills: expressing interest in, partnership with, and commitment to the patient; recognizing, understanding, and responding to patient and physician feelings; being supportive, nonjudgmental, and nondefensive; using nonverbal communication; appropriately using self-disclosure
- Using patient education skills: assessing patient's knowledge, beliefs, needs; tailoring education to needs; giving verbal information (avoiding jargon; categorizing information; being brief, clear, and explicit; using dialogue rather than monologue); providing written instructions; using printed materials; checking patient's comprehension and agreement
- Conducting organized and efficient visits: reviewing the chart before seeing the patient; establishing an agenda and time limits with the patient; prioritizing; focusing on one topic at a time; avoiding premature education; using smooth transitions; summarizing; logically bridging to next visit and negotiating follow-up appointment

Evaluation of a patient's psychosocial status:
- Obtaining a social/psychological history
- Performing a mental/psychological status examination
- Developing a multiaxial diagnostic formulation that includes patient problems (medical and psychosocial), personality characteristics, psychosocial stressors, premorbid and present functional status

Step 4: Educational Strategies

Because the faculty chose to emphasize the attainment of psychomotor (skill) objectives, *experiential learning strategies* are integral to the rotation. Cognitive and attitudinal objectives are addressed through targeted readings and discussions during related experiential learning exercises. *Multiple educational strategies* are used to teach and reinforce learning in most areas. For example, patient education skills are addressed in syllabus readings; in a role-playing and discussion exercise that includes a review of a demonstration videotape; in simulated patient exercises, including one with a noncompliant patient; in observation of a practicing internist who uses these skills; and perhaps in a video review and discussion of the educational segment of an interaction with a patient from the resident's clinic (the resident chooses the focus for video reviews).

Content	The content of the curriculum relates directly to the above listed objectives and is provided in a course syllabus and videotape.
Educational Methods	*Orientation Meeting:* To help faculty and residents get to know one another, to have residents reflect on their learning needs and goals, to convey explicit overall goals and responsibilities for the rotation, and to orient residents to the schedule for the month.
	Syllabus/Readings: Provides a schedule of curriculum events and other practical information, such as locations and directions; defines specific learning objectives in 15 content areas; and provides required and elective readings (handouts or published chapters/articles) for each content area.
	Demonstration/Observation: Demonstration videotape of less- and more-skilled approaches to data gathering, emotion-handling/relationship-building, and patient education used during role-playing sessions. Residents observe one real-life session of a general internist faculty member integrating the various skills as he sees patients in an outpatient setting. Residents gain firsthand experience of resources that they can use during the remainder of their residency by attending Alcoholics Anonymous, Narcotics Anonymous, and Home Care meetings with a faculty facilitator.
	Discussion: Facilitated discussion is part of all experiential learning exercises in order to promote the resident's development of self-awareness, accurate self-assessment, elicitation of feedback, understanding of the material being discussed, and definition of personal learning objectives. Emphasis is placed on creating a positive, safe, and supportive learning environment.
	Didactic Lecture/Discussion: A minilecture/discussion on multiaxial diagnosis, psychosocial history, and mental status examination precedes the experience on the consultation-liaison psychiatry service. There are also minilectures/discussions on the diagnosis and management of anxiety disorders, depressive disorders, and somatoform disorders. Sessions immediately before each of their

general medicine ambulatory continuity clinics address integrating learned skills into ongoing patient care, organizing office visits, utilizing available resources, and maintaining primary care records.

Role-Plays: Used in two to three-hour sessions on data gathering/ agenda setting, emotion handling/relationship building, patient education and compliance, smoking cessation counseling, and alcoholism screening and counseling. Sessions also include discussion, self-assessment, elicitation and receipt of feedback from faculty and fellow residents, and review of learnings/plans for the future.

Simulated Patients: Eight sessions of two to three hours are used to give residents supervised practice in the integrated use of interviewing skills, to teach office psychotherapy skills, and to provide supervised experience in the biopsychosocial diagnosis and management of patients with specific problems. The problems include adjustment reaction; noncompliance; alcoholism in a patient presenting with physical complaints; somatoform disorder; and a primary physical disorder masquerading as a primary psychological disorder. Sessions include discussion of the multiaxial diagnosis of the specific patient; formulation of a biopsychosocial approach to management; self-assessment of skill use and the results; elicitation and receipt of feedback from the patient, fellow residents, and faculty; and review of learnings/plans for the future.

Real-Patient Experience: Residents perform initial evaluations of patients referred for psychiatric evaluation from medical and surgical services. The patient is then seen with the attending consultation-liaison psychiatrist, diagnosis and disposition are discussed, and the consultation note is written collaboratively. In this manner residents gain experience in the evaluation of depressive syndromes (40% of patients), delirium and dementia (20%), personality disorders (10%), and a variety of other psychiatric problems, including anxiety and somatoform disorders. Residents also see and videotape interactions with patients in their own Medical House Staff Practice (two sessions per week).

Video Reviews: During three one-hour sessions with a faculty facilitator, residents review selected videotapes of real or simulated patient encounters.

Role Models: Faculty include general internists in addition to behavioral scientists. Residents observe a faculty internist in his general internal medicine practice (see above). The internists' own clinical experiences often enter the discussions during the above described learning sessions.

Tailoring of Content and Methods to Individual Learners: Ongoing self-assessments, discussions, and faculty observations during the various learning sessions described above provide faculty with a good understanding of residents' learning styles and needs. Sessions are generally flexible enough for faculty to address individual needs within the sessions. Occasionally faculty will meet during a rotation to discuss a coordinated approach to learners with special needs or learners who present difficulties for specific faculty.

Self-Assessment: As described above, before eliciting or receiving feedback from others, residents are asked to assess their own performance after each role-play and simulated patient experience. They are often coached to describe what they did well, as well as to identify what they would like to have done differently and what they would like help with. At the beginning of most experiential learning sessions, residents are asked to identify the skills on which they would like to work and receive feedback. In addition, residents rate themselves relative to the accomplishment of curricular objectives at the beginning and end of the rotation.

Independent Learning Projects: Each resident is required to identify a specific content area, related learning objectives, and appropriate learning resources. Residents are provided with time to pursue independent learning in this area, which usually involves reading; direct observation or experience with the content; reflection; and/or discussion. They describe their experience and learning during a three-hour sign-out with the course coordinator.

Step 5: Implementation

This ambitious and innovative curriculum (at the time of its inception in the early 1980s) required careful planning, anticipation and address of barriers, considerable resources, external funding, faculty development, coordination of multiple faculty and staff, complicated scheduling, and a strategy that would permit mistakes and would encourage ongoing cycles of improvement.

Resources (for each month of operation)	*Personnel*
	▪ Faculty: 0.5 FTE behavioral scientist, who serves as coordinator for planning, scheduling, training of simulated patients, and evaluation, and as facilitator of orientation, four simulated patient office psychotherapy sessions per resident, one role-playing session, video review sessions, and the residents' self-directed learning projects; 0.2 FTE general internist facilitator for two role-playing sessions, three simulated patient sessions, two to three clinic observation and planning sessions; 0.1 FTE additional faculty (behavioral scientist and general internist) for facilitation of smoking cessation and alcoholism sessions; 0.3 FTE psychiatrist who teaches, supervises, and makes rounds with residents on the consultation-liaison psychiatry service. Faculty development during the first few years involved behavioral scientist–internist coteaching, which increased faculty time.

- Simulated patients: 24 to 29 hours per month of the rotation.
- Support staff: 0.1 FTE secretary for scheduling, producing and distributing syllabi, coordinating and paying simulated patients, collecting evaluation forms, and coordinating correspondence related to the course.
- Residents: One month of each resident's time; two to three residents per month.

Facilities: One examining and viewing room equipped with built-in videotaping and viewing capabilities; conference room equipped with a portable videotaping and viewing unit.

Funding: Partial salary support, and funding for simulated patients, comes from a federal grant for generalist residency training; other support is provided by the hospital and the faculty practice group from clinical revenues.

Support

External Support: Faculty and curriculum in this area are required by a federal grant that provides partial funding for the GIM residency program (Bureau of Health Professions, Health Resources and Services Administration). External grant support has been obtained for all but two years of the program's existence.

Internal Support
- Department chair: Evaluations and example videotapes were shared with the department chair during the first few years of the curriculum. As a result, the curriculum was expanded in 1983 to include traditional track as well as GIM track residents.
- Resident support: Residents perceive the rotation as valuable. Their support helped maintain the curriculum and its associated faculty when the GIM residency program temporarily lost federal funding from 1988 to 1990.
- Hospital and faculty: The Med-Psych rotation is an integral part of the hospital's GIM residency program, which has gained a national reputation for its training of generalists and for ongoing curriculum development. The program and its faculty are important in attracting excellent candidates to the residency program and in attracting external funding.

Administration

Administrative Structure: A faculty coordinator, supported by a secretary/administrative assistant, is responsible for planning, implementation, and evaluation of the curriculum.

Communication: The coordinator meets with involved faculty to plan any revisions in the curriculum. Monthly meetings, during which the faculty internist, psychiatrist, and behavioral scientist/ curriculum coordinator complete final evaluations of individual residents, also serve a coordination function. Copies of minutes from the orientation meeting, which provide information on the background and interests of each resident, and from the sign-out meeting, which provide feedback on residents' perceptions of the month, are distributed to all faculty members. Formal evaluation results are distributed yearly. Curriculum objectives and expectations are conveyed to the residents in writing in the syllabus and in person during learning sessions.

Operations: The secretary/administrative assistant, under the direction of the curriculum coordinator, puts together and distributes the schedule of learning sessions and the course syllabus. She ensures that evaluations and self-assessments are collected from the residents. She schedules and pays the simulated patients and maintains the relevant financial records.

Barriers

Resident/Faculty Resistance: In 1979, the curriculum developers expected some resident and faculty resistance to the introduction of psychosocial training into an internal medicine residency training. Having a funded external mandate was helpful in countering any institutional resistance to freeing up curricular time. To counter resident resistance, the curriculum was introduced initially to interested residents (see below). Anticipated resident resistance to role-playing was addressed through facilitation techniques that elicited previous resident experiences with the technique, acknowledged discomfort and artificiality, and provided a safe and supportive learning environment (see Chapter 6). Occasional resident responses that interfered with learning early in the history of the rotation, such as excessive defensiveness and withdrawal after receiving direct feedback on performance, led to changes in facilitator behaviors and amelioration of the problem (7).

Faculty Inexperience: The behavioral scientist faculty for the rotation, while experienced in the teaching of communication skills and psychiatry, were not experienced in the practice of internal medicine. The internal medicine faculty were interested but inexperienced in teaching interviewing skills and the content of the curriculum. During the initial years, the curriculum was cotaught by behavioral scientists and internists who taught one another. The faculty also attended external courses and activities that enhanced their teaching/facilitation skills.

Ineffective Curricular Components: Ongoing evaluation, which included systematic feedback from residents and faculty, as well as summative evaluation results, was used to drive revisions that have strengthened the curriculum, such as attention to the organization and efficiency of office visits, the elimination of unnecessary didactic sessions, and increases in clinically relevant experiential learning.

Introduction

Phase-In: The curriculum was introduced initially to interested GIM track residents who chose the program knowing that such training would be included. This phase-in period permitted time for faculty development and curricular revisions (see above). By 1983, the curriculum was considered so successful that the department contributed additional resources so that the curriculum could be expanded to include all residents.

Step 6: Evaluation

Formative learner and program evaluation are emphasized. Early in the history of the curriculum, quantitative analyses of self-assessments and end of rotation curriculum assessments were performed for summative purposes to assure program effectiveness for the curriculum developers, department chair/residency program director, and the federal agency providing grant funds for the GIM Residency Program. In addition, the faculty conducted a partially funded, focused, randomized, objective assessment of program effectiveness in order to address their own needs for scholarly work and in order to accomplish a more rigorous evaluation of program effectiveness that might be useful to colleagues in other institutions. Consistent with the educational priorities for the rotation, a major focus of the formative and summative evaluation strategies has been the assessment of skill attainment.

Users	Residents, department chair/residency program director, curriculum faculty and coordinators, and professional colleagues.
Uses	Formative information to help the residents achieve learning objectives; formative information to help the faculty improve their individual performances and to help the curriculum coordinator/core faculty improve overall program performance; summative information to help the department chair/residency program director assess individual resident performance and determine program effectiveness/worthiness of continued or increased support; objective summative information that could help professional colleagues from other institutions develop curricula in this area.
Resources	Resources for evaluation have included the following: limited external funds from a federal training grant, an institutional research grant, and a National Institute of Mental Health grant; interested faculty with limited protected academic time; and a colleague from the associated School of Public Health who has research expertise in analyzing doctor–patient interactions
Evaluation Questions	Are learning objectives being achieved by individual residents and by the group of residents who experience the curriculum? What are the strengths of the curriculum? What are its weaknesses? How can the curriculum be improved?
Evaluation Designs	$O_1 - - - X_1 - - - O_2 - - - ... - - - X_{n-1} - - - O_n$ Ongoing self-assessment as well as peer and faculty observation during each experiential learning exercise.

$O_1 - - - X - - - O_2$

There is a self-assessment instrument for program-defined and individual learning objectives.

$X - - - O$

End-of-rotation Department of Medicine evaluation form on each resident which is completed by core Med-Psych faculty; end-of-rotation debriefing with residents; end-of-rotation curriculum evaluation form, which is completed by residents.

E $X - - - O$

R

C $- - - O(- - - X)$

Posttest only randomized controlled evaluation, 1983–86, during which 48 residents were videotaped two months after (or before) completion of the rotation as they interviewed a trained, simulated patient, who was blinded to the pre-post status of the resident.

Evaluation Methods and Instruments	Observation, self-assessment, and feedback are used during experiential learning sessions, sometimes with a communications skills rating form.

Self-assessment instrument on which residents rate the importance and degree of accomplishment of program-defined and individually defined learning objectives, as well as their confidence in diagnosing and treating common psychosocial disorders.

A standard Department of Medicine rating form is completed by faculty at the end of each rotation. It ranks residents on several attribute scales (knowledge; independent learning; gathering of clinical information; quality of consult notes; presentation of clinical data; clinical reasoning ability and judgment; responsibility, initiative, and motivation; organization and efficiency; rapport with patients and family; patient education; relations with co-workers/role as a consultant; humaneness of patient care; ability to take and respond to constructive criticism; integrity; required reading) and asks for written comments on strengths, weaknesses, and areas/suggestions for improvement.

Standard Department of Medicine elective/specialty evaluation rotation forms were completed by residents from 1983 to 1987.

During end-of-rotation meetings with residents, the curriculum coordinator assesses residents' perceptions of rotation, its strengths, its weaknesses, and suggestions for improvement. A typed summary of the meeting is distributed to core faculty and is filed for end-of-year review.

End-of-rotation curriculum assessment forms are completed by residents. These forms elicit ratings of and comments on readings and other curricular components.

From 1983 to 1986, interactions between a trained simulated patient and a resident were videotaped for evaluation purposes before, or two months after, the rotations. Evaluation included: a process and content analysis of the videotapes; simulated patient's ratings of the interaction, and an analysis of the visit note recorded by the resident. The simulated patient and coders were blinded to the pre/post status of the resident.

Ethical Concerns

Standard Department of Medicine rating forms are maintained in the resident's file. The information is considered confidential; access is limited to the resident and responsible faculty. Curriculum assessment forms are completed anonymously by the residents, to encourage candid assessments and to prevent the faculty from being influenced by residents' assessments of the curriculum when the faculty complete the end-of-rotation rating forms for each resident. Evaluation material from the randomized controlled evaluation, which included analysis of each individual resident's interaction with only one simulated patient, was considered appropriate for program (pooled resident) evaluation, but not for individual resident evaluation. This material, therefore, was used for summative program but not summative individual evaluation. The randomized controlled evaluation was designed in a manner that did not withhold the curriculum from control residents.

Data Collection

To the extent possible, evaluation activities are integrated into the curriculum schedule. The secretary ensures that self-assessment and end-of-rotation curriculum assessment forms are completed and returned by the last day of the rotation. If necessary, time is made in the resident's schedule to complete the evaluations before the end of the rotation debriefing meeting.

Data Analysis

Pre-post self-assessments are reviewed by the curriculum coordinator. Tallied summaries of the curriculum-specific assessment forms and the end-of-rotation meeting summaries are reviewed at the end of each year. Analysis of the tallied self-assessment results from 1985 to 1986 revealed significant perceived progress by residents in the achievement of program-defined learning objectives from the beginning to the end of the rotation. Analysis of tallied rotation evaluation forms from 1983 to 1987 revealed that the med-psych rotation compared very favorably to elective/specialty focused rotations. Trained coders were hired to analyze the interactions between residents and the evaluation-simulated patient that were videotaped from 1983 to 1986 and to analyze the recorded notes from the visits. Statistical analysis was performed by a colleague from the School of Public Health. Results revealed that trained residents were more skilled than untrained residents in their use of interviewing skills and tended toward more appropriate management of the patient. There was no significant difference between groups in charting practices.

| Reporting of Results | During the first several years of the rotation, evaluation results were shared with the department chair. Analyses of summative program evaluations have been reported in two separate publications (7, 9). |

Because quantitative analyses of self-assessments revealed similar results from year to year and required time and energy, they were discontinued, although the data are entered into a computer and are accessible if needed. The self-assessments are reviewed with respect to individual learners by the curriculum coordinator and are felt to be part of the learner-centered, self-directed approach to learning that is emphasized in the rotation.

Although the randomized controlled evaluation demonstrated significant differences in the use of interviewing skills between trained and control residents, the trend toward more appropriate management by trained residents did not achieve statistical significance. In retrospect, the case used for evaluation appeared to have been too difficult for many PGY-1 residents and should have been more thoroughly piloted before use. To accurately assess changes in diagnostic and management skills, it would have been preferable to have included several different simulated patient interactions, but there were insufficient resources for such an approach.

Curriculum Maintenance and Enhancement

The curriculum coordinator fulfills important roles in (a) maintaining an ongoing understanding of the curriculum, its faculty and its learners; (b) coordinating changes in the curriculum in response to evaluation results, evolving needs, and changes in available resources; and (c) sustaining the curriculum team through processes of communication, involvement, meetings, and celebrations. The division has encouraged faculty members to participate in related activities that promote continued development as educators and scholars and to network with colleagues with similar interests beyond the institution. The division has also developed programs that are complimentary to the med-psych curriculum.

Understanding the Curriculum	The curriculum coordinator maintains a good understanding of the curriculum through involvement in the evaluation process, review of all evaluation results, and formal and informal meetings with residents and faculty.
Management of Change	Minor operational changes, such as adjustments in a resident's schedule, are made by the curriculum coordinator. Fundamental changes in the curriculum, such as changes in the syllabus or experiential learning exercises, are made by a group of core faculty, consisting of the behavioral scientist (who also serves as the curriculum coordinator), two internists, and the consultation-liaison psychiatrist.
Sustaining the Curriculum Team	During the first several years of the curriculum, faculty development occurred and interest was maintained through a process of coteaching of experiential learning sessions. Currently, faculty

meet periodically to discuss or evaluate individual learners, to review evaluation results, and to revise curricular components. The recognition of individual learner accomplishments is motivating to faculty and sometimes is best appreciated in these meetings, where faculty experiences can be shared. Core faculty have a yearly luncheon meeting with the simulated patients to thank them for their contributions to the program, to elicit their perceptions of how the year went and their suggestions for changes, and to communicate program results and anticipated changes. Minutes from the orientation and end-of-rotation meetings with residents are shared with all faculty members.

Related Activities That Strengthen the Curriculum	*Faculty Development:* Faculty participate in related external faculty development courses and training programs, such as the ones sponsored by the American Academy on Physician and Patient. Med-psych faculty have also developed, participated in, and served as facilitators for the Johns Hopkins Faculty Development Program for Clinician-Educators. Many of the residents' clinical preceptors have been trained in the latter program, which includes a module on interviewing skills.
	Networking/Scholarly Activity: Networking with colleagues who are from other institutions and who have similar interests has resulted in the integration of new teaching techniques, such as the development of the skill-based role-plays described above, and the use of methods to help residents identify and discuss unrecognized behavioral responses and feelings during interviews with patients. Networking has also led to scholarly work related to the evaluation of our own program (9), the development of block curricula in this area for residents (10), the development and evaluation of continuing education in this area for practicing physicians (11), and a study of personal growth in relation to professional growth (in process).

Dissemination

Dissemination activities have forced faculty to evaluate critically and refine their own teaching and educational strategies. The activities have led to networking with colleagues at other institutions. The activities have benefited the med-psych curriculum in terms of additions and improvements; med-psych faculty members in terms of professional growth and promotion; clinical preceptors in our residency program; and colleagues and curricula at other institutions.

Target Audience	The target audiences are (a) faculty who are clinician educators with similar interests at other institutions and (b) faculty with administrative responsibility at home and other institutions.
Reasons for Dissemination	Help address the health care problem defined in Step 1, prevent redundant work, and stimulate change at other institutions.

Promote feedback and interchange/collaboration with colleagues at other institutions. Help curriculum developers achieve recognition and academic advancement.

Content	Literature review problem identification and general needs assessment, at the request of the journal editor as part of the description of the curriculum.

Description of the curriculum.

Guidelines/approaches to designing block curricula (multi-institutional effort).

Curricular materials.

Evaluation results.

Methods	*Workshops* on teaching methods at regional and national professional meetings.

Abstracts on teaching methods and evaluation results at regional and national professional meetings.

Curricular materials (syllabus and demonstration videotape) distributed by direct request or through educational clearing houses.

Articles in peer-reviewed professional journals: Literature review, curriculum description, and some evaluation results (7); randomized controlled evaluation of the curriculum (9); multi-institutionally authored paper on developing block curricula for residents that compares this and two other similar curricula (10).

Faculty Development of GIM Clinical Faculty: module on interviewing skills included in Johns Hopkins Faculty Development for Clinical Educators.

Resources	Semiprotected academic time of some faculty and reimbursement for travel, supported by academic group practice (Johns Hopkins Bayview Physicians, P.A.).

Partial grant support for the randomized, controlled evaluation study (see above, Step 6).

REFERENCES

1. Ende J, Atkins E. Conceptualizing curriculum for graduate medical education. *Acad Med* 1992; 67:528–534.
2. Ende J, Davidoff F. What is curriculum? *Ann Intern Med* 1992; 116:1055–1057.
3. Goroll AH, Morrison G, project codirectors. *Core Medicine Clerkship: Curriculum Guide.* Society of General Internal Medicine and Clerkship Directors in Internal Medicine, Contract No. 240-93-0029, Division of Medicine, Bureau of Health Professions, Health Resources and Ser-

vices Administration, DHHS; U.S. Public Health Service; 1995.

4. ACP Governors' Class of 1996. *Learning from Practitioners: Office-Based Teaching of Internal Medicine Residents.* Philadelphia: American College of Physicians; 1995.

5. Dorman PJ, ed. *Community-Based Teaching: State of the Art and How to Get There.* Proceedings from the National Symposium, Philadelphia, Feb. 2–3, 1996. Philadelphia: Community-Based Teaching Project, American College of Physicians, 1996.

6. American Society of Internal Medicine. *What's So Special about Being an Internist? A "How-to" Resource Kit for Internists on Internal Medicine Preceptorship Programs.* Washington: American Society of Internal Medicine; 1996.

7. Kern DE, Grayson M, Barker LR, Roca RP, Cole KA, Roter D, Golden A. Residency training in interviewing skills and the psychosocial domain of medical practice. *J Gen Intern Med* 1989; 4:421–431.

8. Golden AS. A model for curriculum development linking curriculum with health needs. In Golden AS, Carlson DG, Hogan JL, eds., *The Art of Teaching Primary Care.* New York: Springer Publishing; 1982.

9. Roter DL, Cole KA, Kern DE, Barker LR, Grayson M. An evaluation of residency training in interviewing skills and the psychosocial domain of medical practice. *J Gen Intern Med* 1990; 5:347–354.

10. Williamson P, Smith R, Kern DE, Lipkin Jr. M, Barker LR, Florek J. The medical interview and psychosocial aspects of medicine: Residency block curricula. *J Gen Intern Med* 1992; 7:235–242.

11. Roter DL, Hall JA, Kern DE, Barker LR, Cole KA, Roca RP. Improving physicians' interviewing skills and reducing patients' psychosocial distress: A randomized clinical trial. *Arch Intern Med* 1995; 155:1877–1884.

Additional Resources

Lists of specific and annotated general references appear at the end of each chapter. These lists provide the reader with access to predominantly published resources on curriculum development and evaluation. This appendix supplements the chapter references by providing the reader with a selected list of published and unpublished resources on funding, faculty development, and already developed curricula. If you know of useful resources that have not been included in this list, please write them down on the evaluation sheet at the end of the book and return it to the authors. We will consider them for inclusion in any future editions of the book.

FUNDING RESOURCES

Funds for most medical education programs are provided through the sponsoring institution from tuition, clinical or other revenues or from government support of the educational mission of the institution. External sources that provide direct support for the development, maintenance, and evaluation of specific educational programs are relatively scarce, compared to sources that provide grant support for clinical and basic research. Some government and private entities that do provide direct support for medical education, usually in targeted areas, are listed below.

General Information

- Baumgartner JE, ed. *National Guide to Funding in Health.* 4th ed. Foundation Center, New York; 1995. 1125 pages. This guide is available in medical school libraries. Web site: http://fdncenter.org.
- *The Health Funds Grants Resources Yearbook.* 7th ed. Wall Township, NJ: Health Resources Publishing; 1997. This book includes information on grantmakers' priorities, grantseeking tips, directory of funding resources, and a chapter on health pro-

fessions training. Available from Health Resources Publishing Dept. 1YBK7, 3100 Highway 138, Wall Township, New Jersey 07719-1442; phone: 800-516-4343; fax: 908-681-0490.

Government Resources

- *Guide to Federal Funding for Governments and Nonprofits.* Vols. 1 and 2. 19th ed. Arlington, Virginia, 1997. 1700 pages. This guide is available from Government Information Services, 4301 N. Fairfax Drive, Suite 875, Arlington, Virginia 22203-1627; phone: 800-876-0226 or 703-528-1000; fax: 703-528-6060. $340 plus shipping and handling. Some public libraries and medical school libraries may have this reference.

- The federal government funds *training grants* in the following areas: family medicine for medical students; primary care residency training in family practice, general internal medicine, and pediatrics; faculty development in family medicine, general internal medicine, and pediatrics; podiatry; nursing; and the training of physician assistants. To obtain information on how to apply for a training grant or for a list of currently funded programs, ask for a staff person in "pre-doctoral (medical student) training grants," "residency training grants," "faculty development training grants," "podiatry," "nursing," or "physician assistants" at the following address or phone number:
Health Research Services Administration, Bureau of Health Professions, 5600 Fishers Lane, Room A-27, Rockville, MD 20857. Phone: 301-443-1467.

- For early notification of grant opportunities, try these web sites:
  1. Federal grants: http://www.nih.gov
  2. Agency for Health Care Policy and Research: http://www.ahcpr.gov

Private Foundations

- *Selected list* of foundations that support medical education and health care:
  1. *Josiah Macy, Jr., Foundation:* Josiah Macy, Jr., Foundation Grants, 44 E. 64th Street, New York, NY 10021. Programs, symposiums, conferences, workshops, seminars. Amount: total of approximately $4 million per year. Phone: 212-486-2424.
  2. *Pew Charitable Trusts:* Pew Charitable Trusts Grants, 2005 Market Street, Suite 1700, Philadelphia, PA 19103-7017. Programs: instruction/curriculum development. Amount: $30,000–$300,000 average grants; total per year of approximately $145 million. Phone: 215-575-9050 (for guidelines).
  3. *Robert Wood Johnson Foundation:* Robert Wood Johnson Foundation Grants, Rt. 1 and College Road, East, Princeton, NJ 08543-2316. Programs: service delivery programs; education; research. Amount: total of approximately $260 million per year, with approximately 25% of that total given in grants for education and training. Phone: 609-452-8701.
  4. *Rockefeller Foundation:* Rockefeller Foundation International Grants, Program to Support Science-Based Development, Health Sciences, 120 5th Avenue, New York, NY 10018. Programs: basic research. Amount: total of approximately $9.5 million per year. Phone: 212-869-8500.
  5. *W. K. Kellogg Foundation:* W. K. Kellogg Foundation Grants, P.O. Box 5196, Battle Creek, MI 49016. Programs: instruction/curriculum development; service

delivery programs. Amount: total of $236 million per year. Contact: Manager of Grant Proposals. Phone: 616-968-1611.

- For early notification of grant opportunities, try this web site: http://fdncenter.org

FACULTY DEVELOPMENT RESOURCES

Faculty Development Programs/Courses

Listed below are selected programs, courses, and written resources that address the development of clinician-educators in general and educators for specific content areas.

- *American Academy on Physician and Patient (AAPP):* It offers national and regional faculty development courses for teachers of medical interviewing and psychosocial medicine.
  American Academy on Physician and Patient, Degnon Associates, Inc., 6728 Old McLean Village Drive, McLean, VA 22101. Phone: 703-556-9222; fax: 703-556-8729.

- *American College of Physicians (ACP):* Its Community-Based Teaching Project sponsors symposia and faculty development programs on community-based teaching.
  American College of Physicians, Independence Mall West, 6th Street at Race, Philadelphia, PA 19106-1572. Phone: 800-523-1546.

- *Harvard Macy Institute Program for Physician Educators:* It offers a 19-day in-residence faculty development program, divided into an 11-day winter session and an 8-day spring session. Participants are required to pursue a focused educational project. The program addresses four content areas: learning and teaching; curriculum; evaluation; and leadership.
  Elizabeth G. Armstrong, Ph.D., Office of Educational Development, Harvard Medical School, 260 Longwood Avenue, MEC 384, Boston, MA 02115. Phone: 617-432-0477; fax: 617:734-5224.

- *Johns Hopkins University Faculty Development Program:* It offers nine-month-long, half-day-per-week longitudinal programs in both teaching skills and curriculum development in Baltimore for physicians in the Mid-Atlantic region. Program faculty are also available to consult, develop, and present on-site programs in teaching skills and curriculum development for client institutions in any location.
  Division of General Internal Medicine, Johns Hopkins Bayview Medical Center, 4940 Eastern Avenue, Baltimore, MD 21224. Phone: 410-550-0509; fax: 410-550-3403.
  Teaching Skills Inquiries:
  Longitudinal Programs: Lee Randol Barker, M.D., Sc.M.
  Special Programs: Karan A. Cole, Sc.D.; Penny R. Williamson, Sc.D.
  Curriculum Development Inquiries:
  Longitudinal and Special Programs: Donna M. Howard, Dr.P.H.

- *McMaster University Program for Educational Development and Faculty Development.* It offers a yearly faculty development course in teaching evidence-based medicine.
  Geoff Norman, Ph.D., Program for Educational Development, McMaster University, 1200 Main Street, West, HSC-3N51, Hamilton, Ontario, CANADA L8N 3Z5. Phone: 905-525-9140, ext. 23114.

- *Stanford University Faculty Development Program.* It offers a four-week program in Stanford, California, each summer in each of the following three content areas: principles and skills of clinical teaching, the teaching of medical decision making, the teaching of clinical preventive medicine. Participants agree to return to their home institutions and disseminate what they have learned.
  Kelly Skeff, M.D., Ph.D., or Georgette Stratos, Ph.D., Department of Medicine–S102C, Stanford University Medical Center, Stanford, CA 94305. Phone: 415-725-8802 or 415-725-8807; fax: 415-725-8381.
- *U.S. Public Health Service–Funded Faculty Development Programs.* The U.S. Public Health Service's Bureau of Health Professions, Health Resources and Services Administration funds faculty development programs for primary care–oriented faculty. For a list of currently funded programs, contact the following:
  Health Research Services Administration, Bureau of Health Professions, HRSA, Parklawn Building, Room 9A-27, 5600 Fishers Lane, Rockville, MD 20857. Phone: 301-443-1467.
- *In addition to the above,* individuals may want to contact *professional societies* in their field and *health professional or educational schools* in their area, which may offer faculty development programs or courses.

Written Resources for Faculty Development

- Albright CL. Resources for Faculty Development in Family Violence. *Acad Med* 1997; 72(suppl.):S93–S101.
- American College of Physicians Governor's Class of 1996. *Learning from Practitioners: Office-Based Teaching of Internal Medicine.* Philadelphia: American College of Physicians; 1995. This manual was written by practitioners of internal medicine for potential preceptors. The manual is available from American College of Physicians, phone: 800-523-1546, extension 2600; $10 for ACP members, $13 for non-members.
- American Society of Internal Medicine. *What's So Special about Being an Internist? A Resource Kit for Internists on Internal Medicine Preceptorship Programs.* Washington, DC: American Society of Internal Medicine; 1996. Available from the American Society of Internal Medicine, 2011 Pennsylvania Avenue, NW, Suite 800, Washington, DC 20006; phone: 202-835-2746; fax: 202-835-0443.
- Association of Program Directors in Internal Medicine (APDIM). *Educational Clearinghouse for Internal Medicine: A Peer-Reviewed Compendium of Articles, Books, and Locally Produced Materials for Education in Internal Medicine.* 4th ed. Washington, DC: Association of Program Directors in Internal Medicine. 1996. This is an excellent resource for written materials in 21 educational and curricular topics, including a section on teaching skills development. This resource is available from Educational Clearinghouse for Internal Medicine; phone: 800-622-4558.
- The Clinician-Educator: Resurgence of a tradition. *J Gen Intern Med* 1997; 12(suppl. 2):S1–S110. This supplement contains guidelines for promotion of clinician-educators; articles on an evidence-based approach to keeping up with the medical literature; continuing medical education resources; incorporating research advances into practice; clinical practice guidelines; practical tips on teaching in the outpatient setting; inpatient teaching; strategies for learning and teaching communication and the medical interview; teaching procedural skills; faculty development; in-

stitutional change; recruiting and retaining clinician-educators; career satisfaction; teaching in managed care settings; and the economics of teaching in ambulatory settings.

■ Deutsch SL, Noble J, eds. *Community-Based Teaching: A Guide To Developing Education Programs for Medical Students and Residents in the Practitioners' Offices.* Philadelphia: American College of Physicians; 1997. This resource is available from American College of Physicians, Community-Based Teaching Office, Philadelphia; phone: 215-351-2615.

■ Dewitt TG, Roberts KB, eds. *Pediatric Education in Community Settings: A Manual.* Arlington, VA: National Center for Education in Maternal and Child Health; 1995. (See pp. 124–137.) This manual is available from American Academy of Pediatrics Publications, P.O. Box 747, Elk Grove Village, IL 60009-0747; phone: 800-433-9016; fax: 847-228-1281; $20.

■ Society of Teachers in Family Medicine. *Family Systems Medicine: A Faculty Development Curriculum and Preceptor Education Project (PEP): Workshop Leader's Manual and Workshop.* This resource is available from Society of Teachers in Family Medicine [STFM], 8880 Ward Parkway, Kansas City, MO 64114; phone: 800-274-2237; fax: 816-333-3884.

■ University of Massachusetts Medical Center. *Faculty Development Workbook: Primary Care Futures Project.* This workbook provides teaching modules for developing community faculty. The workbook is available from Area Health Education Center, University of Massachusetts Medical Center, 55 Lake Avenue, North, Worcester, Massachusetts 01655; phone: 508-856-3255; $7.00.

CURRICULAR RESOURCES

Listed below are selected sources of already developed, but often unpublished, curricular materials.

■ *Ambulatory Pediatric Association.* Curricular materials are available in areas such as substance abuse, training residents to serve the underserved, guidelines for residency training, pediatric clerkship curriculum and resource manual, etc. The materials are available from Ambulatory Pediatric Association, 6728 Old McLean Village Drive, McLean VA 22101; phone: 703-556-9222; fax: 703-556-8729.

■ *American Academy on Physician and Patient (AAPP).* This society is dedicated to research, education, and professional standards in doctor–patient communication. The Academy maintains a videotape library; a directory of educational resources on interviewing, interpersonal skills, and psychosocial medicine; an annotated bibliography on doctor–patient communication; and a 50-chapter textbook entitled *The Medical Interview.* It also publishes a quarterly newsletter that serves as a clearinghouse for information on research and education related to the medical interview and psychosocial medicine. For more information, contact the American Academy on Physician and Patient, Degnon Associates, Inc., 6728 Old McLean Village Drive, McLean, VA 22101; phone: 703-556-9222; fax: 703-556-8729.

■ *American Association of Medical Colleges Curriculum Directory and the National Curriculum Database Project* (which supplements and may eventually replace the *Curriculum Directory*). The *Directory* has systematically reported information about medical school curricula since 1970. It is available from American Association of

Medical Colleges, Suite 369, 2450 N Street, NW, Washington, DC 20037; phone: 202-828-0400; no charge to medical schools.

- *Association of Program Directors in Internal Medicine (APDIM), Educational Clearinghouse for Internal Medicine.* Latest edition was October 1996. Booklet is free of charge. There is a modest charge for copies of some documents listed in the booklet. To order, contact Educational Clearinghouse for Internal Medicine, 700 Thirteenth Street, NW, Suite 250, Washington, DC 20005-3960; phone: 800-622-4558 or 202-393-1658; fax: 202-783-1347; E-mail: 70560.154@compuserve.com; web page: www.pitt.edu/leff/apdim

- Dewitt TG, Roberts KB, eds. *Pediatric Education in Community Settings: A Manual.* Arlington, Virginia: National Center for Education in Maternal and Child Health; 1995. (See pp. 124–137). This is a faculty development resource that also contains several examples of sections of curricula for trainees. This resource is available from American Academy of Pediatrics Publications, P.O. Box 747, Elk Grove Village, IL 60009-0747; phone 800-433-9016; fax: 847-228-1281; $20.

- FCIM (Federated Council of Internal Medicine) Task Force on Internal Medicine Residency Curriculum. *Graduate Education in Internal Medicine: A Resource Guide to Curriculum Development.* Ende J, Kelly M, Ramsey P, Sox H, eds. Philadelphia: American College of Physicians; 1997. This resource is available from American College of Physicians, P.O. Box 7777, Philadelphia, PA 19175-1140; phone (credit card only) 800-523-1546, ext. 2600 or 215-351-2600 (M–F, 9–5 ET); fax (credit card only) 215-351-2799, 24 hours per day.

- Goroll AH, Morrison G, project codirectors. *Core Medicine Clerkship: Curriculum Guide.* Society of General Internal Medicine and Clerkship Directors in Internal Medicine, Contract No. 240-93-0029, Division of Medicine, Bureau of Health Professions, Health Resources and Services Administration, DHHS; U.S. Public Health Service, 1995. (This guide is available from Society of General Internal Medicine, 700 Thirteenth Street, NW, Suite 250, Washington, DC 20005; phone: 800-822-3060; fax: 202-783-1347.)

- Noble J, Bithony W, MacDonald P, Thane M et al. The core content of a generalist curriculum for general internal medicine, family practice, and pediatrics. *J Gen Intern Med* 1994; 9(suppl. 1):S31–S42. The authors analyze the educational content of the curricula for teaching the generalist disciplines of pediatrics, internal medicine, and family practice. This article maintains that there is a need to learn both the content of medicine and the skills and attitudes that lie outside factual information and that relate to decision making, communication, and community-based knowledge.

- *Society of General Internal Medicine.* This society offers annual meeting precourses, workshops, task force groups, and a monthly journal on a variety of topics, including teaching curricula/programs directed toward medical students, residents, practicing physicians, and patients. Curricular materials are available in substance abuse, the third-year medicine clerkship, and other areas. Contact Society of General Internal Medicine, Suite 250, 700 Thirteenth Street, NW, Washington, DC 20005; phone: 800-822-3060 or 202-393-1662; fax: 202-783-1347.

- *Society of Teachers in Family Medicine.* Curricula are available in sports medicine, substance abuse, clinical nutrition, innovative primary care curricula for first- and second-year medical students, third-year family medicine clerkship, and other areas. For more information, contact Society of Teachers in Family Medicine (STFM), 8880 Ward Parkway, Kansas City, MO 64114; phone: 800-274-2237.

- *In addition to the above,* individuals may want to contact *professional societies* in the relevant field, which may maintain curricular guidelines, clearinghouses, examples or other resources helpful in developing specific curricula.
- The *Internet* may become a source of information about already developed curricula.

Index

Evaluation Form

**CURRICULUM DEVELOPMENT FOR MEDICAL EDUCATION:
A SIX-STEP APPROACH**

by Kern, Thomas, Howard and Bass

Please take a few minutes to give us feedback on the book. Your suggestions will contribute to future revisions.

1. Please circle degree: M.D.   R.N.   Ph.D.   Other _____
                         Specialty: _____

2. Rate your level of experience in developing curricula prior to reading this book:
       None   Extensive
        1   2   3   4   5

3. Are you currently actively involved in a curriculum development project? (circle)   YES   NO

4. Have you read this book as a **text**? (i.e., Did you read or skim chapters from beginning to end?)
(circle)   YES   NO

5. Have you used this book as a **reference**? (i.e., did you use the index to look up certain topics?)
(circle)   YES   NO

6. Please rate the **usefulness of the content** of this book:

	Not at All Useful			Extremely Useful		Not Read
Examples Given Within Each Chapter	1	2	3	4	5	9
Questions at the End of Each Chapter	1	2	3	4	5	9
Introduction	1	2	3	4	5	9
1. Overview	1	2	3	4	5	9
2. Step 1: Problem Identification and General Needs Assessment	1	2	3	4	5	9
3. Step 2: Needs Assessment of Targeted Learners	1	2	3	4	5	9
4. Step 3: Goals and Objectives	1	2	3	4	5	9

	Not at All Useful			Extremely Useful		Not Read
5. Step 4: Education Strategies	1	2	3	4	5	9
6. Step 5: Implementation	1	2	3	4	5	9
7. Step 6: Evaluation and Feedback	1	2	3	4	5	9
8. Curriculum Maintenance and Enhancement	1	2	3	4	5	9
9. Dissemination	1	2	3	4	5	9
Appendix A. Example Curricula	1	2	3	4	5	9
Appendix B. Additional Resources	1	2	3	4	5	9

7. Rate the conceptual clarity of this book: (circle)

Not at All Clear				Extremely Clear
1	2	3	4	5

8. Rate the degree of "reader friendliness" of the format used in this book (degree to which format facilitated your reading of the book):

Not at All				Very High Degree of Reader Friendliness
1	2	3	4	5

9. Would you recommend this book to others?
_____ No
_____ Yes, as a satisfactory book
_____ Yes, as a good book
_____ Yes, as an outstanding book

10. What are the strengths of this book?
_____
_____
_____
_____

11. What are the weaknesses of this book?
_____
_____
_____
_____

12. Suggestions for improving this book:
_____
_____
_____
_____

Please return to: Curriculum Development, Division of General Internal Medicine
Johns Hopkins Bayview Medical Center
4940 Eastern Avenue, Baltimore, MD 21224-2780

THANK YOU FOR YOUR HELP